Down Syndrom

Ahmed S. Nasr
Ahmed L. Aboulnasr
Engy Amin

Down Syndrome Prenatal Screening and Diagnosis

Comprehensive Review

LAP LAMBERT Academic Publishing

Impressum / Imprint

Bibliografische Information der Deutschen Nationalbibliothek: Die Deutsche Nationalbibliothek verzeichnet diese Publikation in der Deutschen Nationalbibliografie; detaillierte bibliografische Daten sind im Internet über http://dnb.d-nb.de abrufbar.

Alle in diesem Buch genannten Marken und Produktnamen unterliegen warenzeichen-, marken- oder patentrechtlichem Schutz bzw. sind Warenzeichen oder eingetragene Warenzeichen der jeweiligen Inhaber. Die Wiedergabe von Marken, Produktnamen, Gebrauchsnamen, Handelsnamen, Warenbezeichnungen u.s.w. in diesem Werk berechtigt auch ohne besondere Kennzeichnung nicht zu der Annahme, dass solche Namen im Sinne der Warenzeichen- und Markenschutzgesetzgebung als frei zu betrachten wären und daher von jedermann benutzt werden dürften.

Bibliographic information published by the Deutsche Nationalbibliothek: The Deutsche Nationalbibliothek lists this publication in the Deutsche Nationalbibliografie; detailed bibliographic data are available in the Internet at http://dnb.d-nb.de.

Any brand names and product names mentioned in this book are subject to trademark, brand or patent protection and are trademarks or registered trademarks of their respective holders. The use of brand names, product names, common names, trade names, product descriptions etc. even without a particular marking in this work is in no way to be construed to mean that such names may be regarded as unrestricted in respect of trademark and brand protection legislation and could thus be used by anyone.

Coverbild / Cover image: www.ingimage.com

Verlag / Publisher:
LAP LAMBERT Academic Publishing
ist ein Imprint der / is a trademark of
OmniScriptum GmbH & Co. KG
Bahnhofstraße 28, 66111 Saarbrücken, Deutschland / Germany
Email: info@lap-publishing.com

Herstellung: siehe letzte Seite /
Printed at: see last page
ISBN: 978-3-659-12149-4

LIST OF CONTENTS

I

- **List Of Abbreviations:**

ACOG	American College of Obstetricians and Gynecologists
AFAFP	Amniotic fluid alpha-fetoprotein
AFP	Alpha- fetoprotein
AFP- L3	Lens-culinaris agglutinin reactive AFP
ART	Assisted reproductive technique
B-hCG	Free beta subunit of human chorionic gonadotrophine
BOH	Bad obstetric history
BPD	Biparital diameter
BUN	Serum Bio chemistry and Fetal Nuchal translucency screening
CA	Chromosomal abnormality
CA- 125	Cancer antigen 125
CEMAT	Canadian multicentre prospective randomized trial
CRL	Crown rump length
CVS	Chorionic Villus Sampling
DHEA	Dehydroepiandrosterone
DIA	Dimeric inhibin –A
DR	Detection rate
DS	Down syndrome
ECEMC	Collaborative study of congenital malformation
FASTER	First and Second Trimester Evaluation Risk
FISH	Fluroescent in situ hybridization
FMF	Frontomaxillary facial angle
FPR	False positive rate
FSH	Follicle stimulating hormone

HCG	Human chorionic gonadotrophine
IDDM	Insulin dependent diabetes mellitus
Inh- A	Dimeric inhibin- A
IVF	In vitro fertilization
LR	Likelihood Ratios
MCA	Multiple congenital anomalies
MCV	Mean corpuscular volume
MI	The first meiotic stage
MII	The second meiotic stage
MoM	Multiple of median
MR	Mental retardation
MRI	Magnatic resonance imaging
MSAFP	Maternal serum alpha- fetoprotein
NBL	Nasal bone length
NHS	National institute for clinical excellance
NSC	National screening committee
NT	Nuchal translucency
NTD	Neural tube defect
OAPR	Odds of being affected given a positive result
OFD	Occipto frontal diameter
PGD	Preimplantation genetics diagnosis
PUBS	Percutaneous umbilical blood sampling
SD	Stander Deviation
SP1	Schwangerschafts protein
SURUSS	Serum, urine and ultrasound screening study
UK-NSC	United kingdom National screening committee

INTRODUCTION

Congenital abnormalities account for 20-25% of perinatal deaths. Now, many genetic and other disorders can be diagnosed early in pregnancy. Prenatal diagnosis uses various noninvasive and invasive techniques to determine the health of, the condition of, or any abnormality in an unborn fetus *(Singh 2005)*.

The risk to any pregnant couple of having a live born infant with a chromosomal abnormality or structural defect is between 3% and 5% *(O'Leary et al., 2006)*.

Definition:

Down syndrome (trisomy 21) is the most commonly recognized genetic cause of mental retardation. The risk of trisomy 21 is directly related to maternal age *(Newberger 2000)*.

Down syndrome is a frequent form of mental retardation associated with characteristic morphologic features (mongolism) and many somatic abnormalities due to a number of chromosomal aberrations *(Dourmishev & Janniger 2003)*.

Down syndrome is a variable combination of congenital malformations caused by trisomy 21. It is the most commonly recognized genetic cause of mental retardation, with an estimated prevalence of 9.2 cases per 10,000 live births in the United States *(Newberger 2000)*.

Because of the morbidity associated with Down syndrome, prenatal screening and diagnostic testing for this condition are offered as optional components of prenatal care. The purpose of prenatal screening and diagnosis is to identify those women at increased risk for an affected pregnancy and to maximize the options available to their families *(Benn 2002).*

Prenatal diagnosis of trisomy 21 allows parents the choice of continuing or terminating an affected pregnancy *(Newberger 2000).*

In the absence of prenatal diagnosis and therapeutic abortion, the prevalence of Down syndrome in developed countries is 1-2 per 1,000 births making it the most frequent identifiable cause of severe learning difficulty. In 95% of cases there is non-disjunction of chromosome 21; in 4% a translocation and 1% are mosaic *(Cuckle 2005).*

Advanced maternal age is by far the strongest epidemiological variables with birth prevalence increasing from 0.6 to 4.1 per 1,000 between age 15 and 45 there is familial aggregation having had a previous Down syndrome pregnancy confers a risk 4.2 per 1,000 higher risk than the age-specific prevalence Other risk factors are considerably weaker *(Cuckle & Arbuzova 2005).*

Difference between screening and diagnostic tests:

All forms of prenatal testing for Down syndrome must be voluntary. A nondirective approach should be used when presenting patients with options for prenatal screening and diagnostic testing. Patients who will be 35 years or older on their due date should be offered chorionic villus sampling or second-trimester amniocentesis *(David et al., 2000)*.

Women younger than 35 years should be offered maternal serum screening at 16 to 18 weeks of gestation. The maternal serum markers used to screen for trisomy 21 are alpha-fetoprotein, unconjugated estriol and human chorionic gonadotrophin. The use of ultrasound to estimate gestational age improves the sensitivity and specificity of maternal serum screening *(David et al., 2000)*.

Diagnosis has been defined as, the patient has the disease or condition of concern. It tends to be more expensive and require an elaborate procedure *(ACOG 2001)*.

Screening has been defined as, the systematic application of a test to individuals at risk of a specific disorder to benefit from further investigation or direct preventative action, among persons who have not sought medical attention on account of symptoms of the disorder, The goal is to estimate the risk of the patient having the disease or condition *(ACOG 2001)*.

Screening tests are quick and easy to do. However, screening tests have more chances of being wrong. There are "false-positives" test states the patient has the condition when the patient really doesn't have this genetic abnormality and "false-negatives" patient has the condition but the test state doesn't show that *(ACOG 2001)*.

The screening policy for Down syndrome may be divided into three types according to the criteria used to identify pregnancies at increased risk. **First,** maternal age alone. **Second**, first-trimester screening with testing between 8 and 13 weeks gestational age using a combination of maternal age with serum markers and/or ultrasound markers. **Third,** second-trimester screening with testing between 14 and 22 weeks gestational age using a combination of maternal age with serum markers *(Holding 2002)*.

The detection rate of a given false positive tests is a convenient and widely used way of comparing the effectiveness of different screening policies. The performance of Down syndrome screening is usually estimated for a standard population of maternities with a specified age distribution *(Wald & Hackshaw 2000)*.

However, this is the goal of prenatal screening and diagnosis. The goal has been clearly defined by peter Rowley who notes that, the aim of genetic screening programs and prenatal cytogenetic diagnosis should be to maximize the options available to families rather than to reduce the prevalence of genetic diseases. Options will be maximized while minimizing procedure-related losses and costs when risk estimates are based on maternal serum screening before a decision is made regarding amniocentesis *(Egan et al., 2000)*.

CHAPTER 1

DOWN SYNDROME AND CHROMOSOMAL ABERRATIONS

Historical Background:

English physician **John Langdon Down** first characterized Down syndrome as a distinct form of mental retardation. In **1862** and in a more widely published report in **1866,** entitled "Observations on an ethnic classification of idiots". due to his perception that children with Down syndrome shared physical facial similarities (epicanthal folds) with those of Blumenbach's Mongolian race, Down used terms such as *mongolism* and *mongolian idiocy.* Idiocy was a medical term used at that time to refer to a severe degree of intellectual impairment. Down wrote that mongolism represented retrogression, the appearance of Mongoloid traits in the children of allegedly more advanced Caucasian parents *(Burke et al., 2006).*

By the **20th century, "mongolian idiocy** "had become the most recognizable form of mental retardation. Most people with it were institutionalized. Few of the associated medical problems were treated, and most died in infancy or early adult life. With the rise of the eugenics movement, 33 of the 48 United States and a number of countries began programs of involuntary sterilization of individuals with Down syndrome and comparable degrees of disability. The ultimate expression of this type of public policy was the German euthanasia program "Aktion T-4" begun in 1940. Court challenges and public revulsion led to discontinuation or repeal of such programs during the decades after World War II *(Zuckoff 2002).*

5

Until the middle of the 20th century, the cause of Down syndrome remained unknown. Although the presence in all races, the association with older maternal age and the rarity of recurrence had been noticed. Standard medical texts assumed it was due to a combination of inheritable factors which had not been identified. Other theories focused on injuries sustained during birth *(Burke et al., 2006)*.

In **1932**, **Waardenburg** suggested that Down syndrome was a consequence of a chromosomal abnormality "trisomy 21". During the past 50 years, great studies have been made toward understanding and treating the myriad medical condition associated with Down syndrome *(George & Capone 2001)*.

With the discovery of karyotype techniques in the 1950s it became possible to identify abnormalities of chromosomal number or shape. **In 1959, Professor Jérôme Lejeune** discovered that Down syndrome resulted from an extra chromosome. The extra chromosome was subsequently labeled as the 21st and the condition as trisomy 21 *(Lejeune 2006)*.

In **1961**, a group of nineteen geneticists wrote to the editor of *The Lancet* suggesting that mongolian *idiocy* had misleading connotations, had become an embarrassing term and should be changed. *The Lancet* supported *Down syndrome*. The World Health Organization (WHO) officially dropped references to *mongolism* in 1965 after a request by the Mongolian delegate *(Shire 2005)*.

In 1975, the United States National Institute of Health convened a conference to standardize the nomenclature of malformations. They recommended eliminating the possessive form "The possessive use of an eponym should be discontinued, since the author neither had nor owned the disorder." While both the possessive and non-possessive forms are used in the general population, Down syndrome is the accepted term among professionals in the USA, Canada and other countries, while Down syndrome continues to be used in the United Kingdom and other areas *(Buckley 2000)*.

Throughout this century distinct genetic, neurobiological, metabolic, developmental, and medical models of Down syndrome have evolved, each having its own set of principles, pedagogy and practices that has produced a separate definition of reality among basic scientists, health care practitioners, and parents, as well as an array of treatment options both real and imagined *(George & Capone 2001)*.

In the 1960s, eukaryotic cell nuclei were observed to contain linear bodies that were named chromosomes. There are normally two copies of each chromosome (homologous pairs) present in every somatic cell.

Human cells normally have 46 chromosomes, which can be arranged in 23 pairs. Of these 23, 22 are alike in males and females, these are called the autosomes. The 23rd pair is the sex chromosome X and Y.

Human cells divide in two ways. The first is ordinary cell division **mitosis**, by which the body grows. In this method, one cell becomes two cells, which have the exact same number and type of chromosomes as the parent cell.

The second method of cell division occurs in the ovaries and testicles **meiosis** and consists of one cell splitting into two, with the resulting cells having half the number of chromosomes of the parent cell. So, normal eggs and sperm cells only have 23 chromosomes instead of 46 *(Leshin 2003)*.

Chromosomal Aberrations:

Many errors can occur during cell division. In meiosis, the pairs of chromosomes are supposed to split up and go to different spots in the dividing cell; this event is called **disjunction**. However, occasionally one pair doesn't divide, and the whole pair goes to one spot. This means that in the resulting cells, one will have 24 chromosomes and the other will have 22 chromosomes. This accident is called **nondisjunction.** If a sperm or egg with an abnormal number of chromosomes merges with   a normal mate, the resulting fertilized egg will have an abnormal number of chromosomes.

The number of chromosomes per cell is unique and characteristic for each species and increasing or decreasing the genetic material produces chromosomal aberrations. Chromosomal aberrations are either **numerical** or **structural** and may involve one or more autosome, Sex chromosomes or both. A given abnormality may be present in all body cells or there may be two or more cell lines; the latter situation is termed mosaicism *(Leshin 2003).*

Robertsonian translocation:

The extra chromosome 21 material that causes Down syndrome may be due to a Robertsonian translocation in this case. The long arm of chromosome 21 is attached to another chromosome, often chromosome 14 (45, XX, t (14; 21q)) or itself called an isochromosome (45, XX, t (21q; 21q)). The manner by which this occurs is through a parent with a balanced translocation. The balanced translocation figure shows a 14/21 translocation, where the other chromosomes are not shown. The individual has two copies of everything on chromosome 14, and two copies of all of the material on the long arm of chromosome 21(21q).
The individual only has one copy of the material on the short arm of chromosome 21(21p), but this appears to have no discernable effect. Individuals with this chromosomal arrangement are phenotypically normal.

During meiosis, the chromosomal arrangement interferes with normal separation of chromosomes. Possible gametic arrangements are: Normal 14 and normal 21; Translocated 14/21 and normal 21; translocated 14/21 only; Normal 14 and translocated 14/21; Normal 21 only. When combined with a normal gamete from the other parent, the last two are lethal, leading to spontaneous abortion. The first, combined with a normal gamete from the other parent, gives rise to a normal child. The second, leads to a translocation Down syndrome child **(Fig. 1)**. The third becomes a translocation carrier, like the parent.

Translocation Down syndrome is often referred to as familial *Down syndrome*. It is the cause of 2-3% of the observed Down syndromes. It does not show the maternal age effect and is just as likely to have come from fathers as mother *(Burke et al., 2006)*.

Mosaicism:

Mosaic Down syndrome is when some of the cells in the body are normal and some cells have trisomy 21, an arrangement called a **mosaic** (46 XX / 47 XX, 21).This can occur in one of two ways: A nondisjunction event during an early cell division leads to a fraction of the cells with trisomy 21 or a Down syndrome embryo undergoes nondisjunction and some of the cells in the embryo revert back to the normal chromosomal arrangement. There is considerable variability in the fraction of trisomy 21, both as a whole and tissue-by-tissue. This is the cause of 1-2% of the observed Down syndromes. There is evidence that mosaic Down syndrome may produce less developmental delay, on average, than full trisomy 21 *(Burke et al., 2006)*.

Duplication of a portion of chromosome 21:

Rarely, a region of chromosome 21 will undergo a duplication event. This will lead to extra copies of some but not all of the genes on chromosome 21 [46, XX, dup (21q)]. If the duplicated region has genes that are responsible for Down syndrome physical andmental characteristics, such individuals will show those characteristics. This cause is very rare and no rate estimates are possible *(Burke et al., 2006)*.

10

Fig. (1): Karyotype of male with trisomy 21 *(Leshin 2003)*.

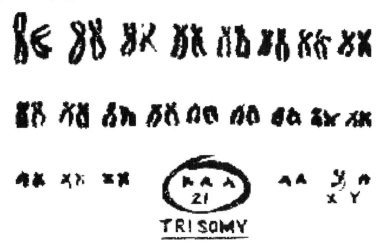

Chromosomal Nondisjunction and Maternal Age:

Researchers have established that the likelihood that a reproductive cell will contain an extra copy of chromosome 21 increases dramatically as a woman ages. Therefore, an older mother is more likely than a younger mother to have a baby with Down syndrome. However, of the total population older mothers have fewer babies about 75% of babies with Down syndrome are born to younger women, because more younger women than older women have babies only about 9% of total pregnancies occur in women 35 years or older each year, but about 25% of babies with Down syndrome are born to women in this age group *(Wellesley et al., 2002)*.

It has been estimated that at least 30 % of oocytes in women aged > 40 years have undergone non-disjunction. The reason for the correlation between late maternal age and non-disjunction is unknown. It is thought to be due to some aspects of aging of the oocyte, which lives in suspended animation during meiotic division from fetal life until that oocyte participates in ovulation.

In addition the mitochondrial ageing hypothesis would explain the relationship between maternal age and the frequency of trisomes e.g. Down syndrome. It was postulated that as a women ages, DNA mutations accumulates in her oocytes, and that the frequency of aneuploidy increases *(Schon et al., 2000)*.

Based on the fact that oocytes require high concentrations of ATP *(Van Blerkom & Runner, 1984; Van Blerkom, 1991)* and the accumulation of DNA mutations have harmful effects on mitochondrial energy production and on overall

12

energy levels in the oocytes, the percentage of chromosomal nondisjunction increases with ageing *(Schon et al., 2000)*.

Also DNA mutations that accumulate over time in the surrounding follicular cells might also lead to aneuploidy *(Schon et al., 2000)*.

The incidence of Down syndrome rises with increasing maternal age. Many specialists recommend that women who become pregnant at age 35 or older undergo prenatal testing for Down syndrome. The likelihood that a woman under 30 who becomes pregnant will have a baby with Down syndrome is less than 1 in 1,000, but the chance of having a baby with Down syndrome increases to 1 in 400 for women who become pregnant at age 35. The likelihood of Down syndrome continues to increase as a woman ages, so that by age 42, the chance is 1 in 60 that a pregnant woman will have a baby with Down syndrome, and by age 49, the chance is 1 in 12. But using maternal age alone will not detect over 75% of pregnancies that will result in Down syndrome *(NICHD 2007)*.

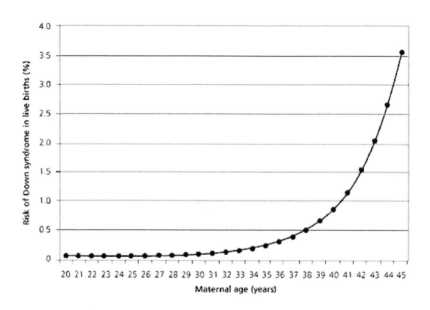

Fig. (2): Chromosomal Nondisjunction and Maternal Age *(Newberger 2000).*

14

Chromosome 21:

Chromosome 21, the smallest human autosome, contains 33.8 million base pairs of DNA and is found to contain only about 250 genes rather than the previously suspected 500-1000. Many or all of which contribute to the pathogenesis and phenotype of Down syndrome *(Hattori et al., 2000)*.

Chromosome 21 is acrocentric, with two arms (21p and 21q) and its centromere close to one end as shown in **(Fig. 3)**. The short arm (21p) do not seems to be essential for normal development, because duplications or deletions in this region usually have few observable phenotypic manifestations. All of the other genes on the chromosome 21 map to the long arm (21q).

Several studies tried to determine which regions of chromosome 21 are involved in the pathogenesis of specific features of Down syndrome **(Epstein *et al.*, 1991; Delabar *et al.*, 1993)**. Functional analysis of newly identified developmental regulated genes that map to the Down syndrome locus may help provide information about the cellular and molecular basis of mental retardation in Down syndrome *(McKusick 1999)*.

Trisomy 21 is the most common autosomal aneuploidy compatible with postnatal survival. It occurs 1 in 800 to 1000 live births in all ethnic groups. Trisomy 21 usually results from nondisjunction in meiosis, most frequently in meiosis I.

Trisomy 21 is the cause of approximately 95% of observed Down syndromes, with 88% coming from nondisjunction in the maternal gamete and 8%

coming from nondisjunction in the paternal gamete.Mitotic nondisjunctions after conception would lead to mosaicism *(Hassold & Sherman 2000)*.

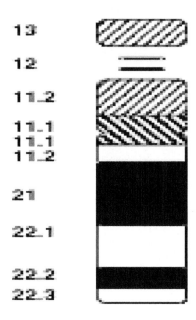

Fig. (3): Chromosome 21 *(Patterson 1995)*

Etiology and Clinical Manifestations of Down syndrome:

Down syndrome is usually identified soon after birth by a characteristic pattern of dysmorphic features **(Table 1)**. The diagnosis is confirmed by karyotype analysis. Trisomy 21 is present in 95% of persons with Down syndrome. Mosaicism, a mixture of normal diploid and trisomy 21 cells, occurs in 2%. The remaining 3% have a Robertsonian translocation in which all or part of an extra chromosome 21 is fused with another chromosome. Most chromosome-21 translocations are sporadic. However, some are inherited from a parent who carries the translocation balanced by a chromosome deletion.

Molecular genetic studies reveal that 95% of occurrences of trisomy 21 result from nondisjunction during meiotic division of the primary oocytes. The exact mechanism for this meiotic error remains unknown. Most trisomy 21 pregnancies prove to be nonviable. Only one quarter of fetuses with trisomy 21 survive to term.

Persons with Down syndrome usually have mild to moderate mental retardation. In some, mental retardation can be severe. School-aged children with Down syndrome often have difficulty with language, communication and problem-solving skills. Adults with Down syndrome have a high prevalence of early Alzheimer's disease, further impairing cognitive function. A number of congenital malformations and acquired diseases occur with increased frequency in persons with Down syndrome. Congenital heart disease and pneumonia are leading causes of mortality, especially in early childhood *(Newberger 2000)*.

Down syndrome involving total trisomy 21 results from nondisjunction, usually in formation of the eggs or sperm, where a gamete ends up with an extra chromosome 21. Nondisjunction may occur in the first meiotic stage (MI) or the second meiotic stage (MII). The extra chromosome 21 is of maternal origin in 80-93 % of the cases and of paternal origin in 7-20% of the cases. Among trisomy 21 cases of maternal origin, approximately 75% result from nondisjunction in meiotic I and 25% in meiotic II while 40% of trisomy 21 cases of paternal origin occur from nondisjunction in meiotic I and 60 % from nondisjunction in meiotic II *(Jyothy et al., 2001; Muller et al., 2000; Antonarakis, 1998; Savage et al., 1998; Yoon et al., 1996; Antonarakis et al., 1992; Buraczynska et al., 1989; Mattei et al., 1979; Magenis et al., 1977)*. There is no maternal age difference between maternal meiotic I and meiotic II nondisjunction *(Antonarakis, 1993; Sherman et al., 1994; Lapunzina et al., 2002)*.

Clinical manifestation:

Children with Down syndrome have a distinct facial appearance. Though not all children with Down syndrome have the same features, some of the more common features are:

- Flattened facial features
- Protruding tongue
- Small head.
- Upward slanting eyes, unusual for the child's ethnic group.
- Unusually shaped ears.

Children with Down syndrome may also have:

- Poor muscle tone
- Broad, short hands with a single crease in the palm

- Relatively short fingers
- Excessive flexibility *(Mayo Clinic 2007)*.

The degree of medical problems and mental retardation varies. Talents, abilities and pace of development differ. People with Down syndrome may be born with or develop:

- Vision problems
- Hearing loss
- Heart defects
- Increased incidence of acute leukemia
- Frequent ear infections and increased susceptibility to infection in general.
- Gastrointestinal obstruction (imperforate anus, and similar problems).
- Esophageal atresia or duodenal atresia
- One third of patients experience blocked airways during sleep.
- At older ages there is an increased incidence of dementia.
- Instability of the back bones at the top of the neck; can result in compression injury of the spinal cord.
- Urinary system defects.
- High blood pressure in the lungs.
- Seizures.
- An under-active thyroid (hypothyroidism).
- Slow growth.
- Late to sit, walk, toilet train.
- Speech problems.
- Obesity.

- Emotional problems.
- Risk that others assume that a child is more retarded than he or she is.

Most of these health problems are treatable and the majority of people born with Down syndrome today have a life expectancy of approximately 55 years *(Frisch 2006)*.

Table (1): Frequency of Dysmorphic Signs in Neonates with Trisomy 21

Dysmorphic sign	Frequency (%)
Flat facial profile	90
Poor Moro reflex	85
Hypotonia	80
Hyperflexibility of large joints	80
Loose skin on back of neck	80
Slanted palpebral fissures	80
Dysmorphic pelvis on radiographs	80
Small round ears	60
Hypoplasia of small finger, middle phalanx	60
Single palmar crease	45

(Newberger 2000)

CHAPTER 2

PRECONCEPTION RISK FACTORS FOR DOWN SYNDROME

With the introduction of a screening test for Down syndrome, genetic screening has been broadened to include women who have not had access to it in the past. Many physicians are offering pregnant women multiple markers testing for Down syndrome between 15 and 20 week's gestation *(Egan et al., 2000).*

1. High maternal age:

Although the risk of Down syndrome is higher in older women, most pregnancies occur in women younger than 35 years and most cases of Down syndrome are missed when screening is restricted to women over 35 *(Egan et al., 2000)*. In England and Wales, prenatal diagnosis of Down syndrome cases rose from 28% in 1989 to 53% in 1999 and the number of invasive tests done to diagnose each case fell significantly *(Bindman et al., 2003).*

Current recommendations from the National Institute for Clinical Excellence are that all pregnant women should be offered a test that provides the current standard of a detection rate of above 60% with a false positive rate of less than 5%. By April 2007 the NHS is required to provide a test that has a detection rate above 75% and a false positive rate of less than 3%. Only the combined, integrated, quadruple and serum integrated tests will meet the more stringent criteria prenatal screening *(Kumar & O'Brien 2004).*

2. Maternal serum markers:

Before the introduction of serum marker testing, most Down syndrome infants were not detected before birth. Screening was based on the increasing risk of Down syndrome with maternal age *(Cate 1999)*. Maternal age and levels of two or more serum analytes maternal serum alpha-fetoprotin [AFP], human chorionic gonadotrophin [hCG] and unconjugated estriol [uE$_3$] are used to calculate a patient-specific risk *(Cate 1999)*.

In *1984 Merkatz et al.* retrospectively analyzed the maternal serum alpha fetoprotein (AFP) in 44 Down affected pregnancies and found it to be low. Subsequently, *Bogart et al., 1987* found elevated levels of maternal serum human chorionic gonadotrophin (hCG) and *Canick et al., 1988* found low levels of unconjugated estriol (uE3) in Down syndrome pregnancies. The reason for these biochemical changes is not yet fully understood but may relate to functional immaturity, leading to a delay in the normal gestational rise or fall *(Pandya 2006)*.

The best combination of maternal serum markers is still debated. Screening performance depends on the combination of markers chosen and whether ultrasound has been used to date the pregnancy accurately. The optimal window for second trimester biochemical screening is between 15 and 22 weeks gestation. Apart from maternal age and gestation, other factors which affect the expected levels of the biochemical markers must be taken into account. These include maternal weight, ethnic origin, the presence of insulin dependent diabetes mellitus, multiple pregnancy, previous Down syndrome pregnancy, smoking and vaginal bleeding *(Pandya 2006)*.

3. Recurrence risk and family history:

If the patient has had a trisomy 21 pregnancy in the past, the risk of recurrence in a subsequent pregnancy increase to approximately 1 percent above the baseline risk determined by the maternal age. Diagnosis of a chromosome-21 translocation in the fetus or newborn is an indication for karyotype analysis of both parents. If both parents have normal karyotypes, the recurrence risk is 2 to 3 percent. If one parent carries a balanced translocation, the recurrence risk depends on the sex of the carrier parent and the specific chromosomes that are fused *(Newberger 2000)*.

The significance of a family history of Down syndrome depends on the karyotype of the affected person (proband). If the proband has trisomy 21, the likelihood of a trisomy 21 pregnancy is minimally increased for family members other than the parents. If the proband has a chromosome-21 translocation or if the karyotype is unknown, family members should be offered genetic counseling and karyotype analysis *(Newberger 2000)*.

4. Previous history of Down syndrome babies:

Most authors considered that young mothers with previous Down syndrome infant had a 1-2% risk of recurrence, while for older mothers this risk is limited to that inherent to maternal age. When a translocation is detected in the parents, the risk of recurrence depends on the type of translocation and on the sex of the carrier parent *(Hecht &Hook 1996)*.

5. Consanguinity:

Consanguinity may result in the homozygous condition for recessive autosomal/deleterious genes. The incidence of consanguinity reported in India 5-60% and uncle-niece and first cousin are the more commonly occurring relation ships in Indian population *(Mueller & Young 2001)*.

It is a well-known fact that consanguinity may increase the chance of individuals having identical genes. The homozygosity may have effect on the clinical conditions such as bad obstetric history [BOH], mental retardation [MR], multiple congenital anomalies [MCA], Down syndrome [DS], primary amenorrhea and primary infertility with suspected genetic etiology. The classified genetic etiologies are the single gene disorders, chromosomal abnormality and multifactorial inheritance. The CA, numerical and structural, may occur as de-novo at post zygotic mitosis or transmitted because of the errors at meiosis in the parental gametogenesis. Consanguinity has been suspected to have its influence in the formation of chromosomal abnormality [CA] *(Amudha et al., 2005)*.

It has been postulated that the high frequency of trisomic syndromes in children, born of young mothers, may be because of non disjunction of chromosomes, in females married to their maternal uncle cousin *(Penrose 1961)*. In India, in a hospital-based study, among consanguineous marriages, a higher frequency of Down syndrome has been noticed. Another study has also observed an increased frequency of parental consanguinity, among the parents of the patients with Down syndrome. Subsequently, one of the studies has failed to confirm a higher incidence of close consanguinity among parents of individuals with Down syndrome *(Amudha et al., 2005)*.

The effect of consanguinity on MR and or multiple congenital malformations has been widely reported. Consanguinity has not influenced the fertility or the prevalence of MCA, CA and genetic disorders, has also been found. However, *Verma et al., 1992* have noticed a significantly higher rate of stillbirths and infant mortality, in consanguinity *(Bittles 2002)*.

A significant frequency has been reported between consanguinity and genetic disorders, congenital heart disease, MCA, neurological malformations, chromosomal disorders and MR *(Jain et al., 1993)*. It has been stated that the association of recessive genetic disorders to consanguinity may be negated by urbanization and the decreased family sizes which predictably will lead to a decline in the consanguinity associated genetic disorders *(Bittles 2002)*.

A sample size of 305 cases with confirmed CA has been studied. Even though, the influence of consanguinity on CA has been observed, it has not been reflected on the types of CA, neither on the numerical nor on the structural CA. The differences may be because of the sample size, the mode of selection and the pooling of the CA as well as the types of consanguinity *(Amudha et al., 2005)*.

The interpretations from the observations of the study are:

1. Consanguinity may have its influence on MCA.
2. One of the genetic etiologies for multiple congenital anomalies is CA.
3. The effect of consanguinity on CA, but not on the types of CA, may be because of its association to MCA rather than to CA. The role of consanguinity is always under speculation *(Amudha et al., 2005)*.

The findings of the study may be interpreted that until and unless definite clinical conditions with CA as the etiology have been known to be associated to the consanguinity; the socioeconomic advantages definitely may outweigh the advocacy against consanguinity especially in India. Hence, it is apparent that at the time of counseling, it may be kept in mind, that consanguinity may have a higher risk than the general population risk on CA *(Amudha et al., 2005)*.

6. <u>Periconceptional Exposure to Contraceptive Pills and Risk for Down syndrome:</u>

Many studies have analyzed the relationship between prenatal exposure to oral contraceptive pills (OCs) and Down syndrome and the results are conflicting.

One of the earliest published studies retrospectively analyzed 10,478 singleton births. Of these, 27% were born to oral contraceptive users, defined as taking OCs in the 3 months before the last menstrual period. The other 73% of patients did not take OCs *(Kasan & Andrew 1985)*. After such factors as age, parity and smoking history were taken into account, there was no significant increase in incidence of Down syndrome in OC users compared with nonusers *(Kandinov 2005)*.

Two studies from Sweden *(Kallen 1989; Ericson et al., 1983)* compared the use of OCs in women with infants with Down syndrome and women who had born normal infants (after stratification for maternal age and parity). Both concluded that there is no association between OC use and Down syndrome.

A case-control study from Spain using data from the Spanish Collaborative Study of Congenital Malformations (ECEMC) found a 2.8-fold increased risk for infants with Down syndrome in women younger than 35 years of age if the mother became pregnant while taking OCs. This risk approaches that for mothers older than 34 years old, which is at risk for Down syndrome secondary to their age by itself, though OC use at the time of conception by women older than 34 years of age did not increase the risk of Down syndrome. The researchers recommended offering prenatal diagnosis for Down syndrome to younger patients who become pregnant while taking oral contraceptive pills *(Frias et al., 2001)*.

Another study *(Yang et al., 1999; Bracken et al., 1978)* examined maternal smoking and use of oral contraceptive pills as possible risk factors for trisomy 21. Although the combined use of cigarettes and OCs increased the risk of Down syndrome (odds ratio =7.62; 95% confidence interval = 1.6-35.6), OC use alone was not a significant risk factor.

Preconception exposures to oral contraceptive pills are overall safe if taken before conception or during the very early stages of pregnancy. There was a suggestion that women who both smoked and used OCs during the pregnancy were more likely to deliver an infant with Down syndrome. Pregnant women older than 35 years of age are routinely offered prenatal testing for Down syndrome. Some researchers recommend prenatal screening for Down syndrome in patients who were taking oral contraceptive pills immediately before pregnancy or even during the very early stages of pregnancy. Although this is definitely a minority view, every case should be managed after weighing all the risks and benefits pertinent to the specific patient *(Kandinov 2005)*.

7. Preconceptional elevated FSH concentrations and risk for Down syndrome:

Due to limited knowledge of pre-conceptional risk factors for trisomy-21 pregnancies, there are currently no pre-conceptional screening tests to identify women at increased risk for a Down syndrome pregnancy *(Wald et al., 1999)*. Recent studies have reported a relation between signs of accelerated depletion of the ovarian reserve and aneuploid pregnancies *(Montfrans et al., 2001)*.

One of them reported that women with history of a Down syndrome pregnancy had significantly elevated follicle stimulating hormone (FSH) concentrations in the early follicular phase of the menstrual cycle *(Montfrans et al., 1999)*.

It was also reported that women who recently had experienced an abortion of a conception with an abnormal karyotype had elevated basal FSH and oestradiol concentrations *(Nasseri et al., 1999)*. Another study reported that women with a reduced ovarian complement (either by surgical removal or congenital absence of one ovary) were more likely to have delivered a child with Down syndrome *(Freeman et al., 2000)*.

The results of these studies suggest that pre-conceptional screening for signs of depletion of the primordial follicle pool could become useful in identifying women at risk for aneuploid pregnancies. However, when elevated basal FSH concentrations are identified during subfertility evaluation, subfertile patients who achieve pregnancy theoretically are exposed to a 2.8-increased risk for a Down syndrome pregnancy *(Montfrans et al., 2001)*.

28

Although two separate studies have reported a relation between aneuploid pregnancies and elevated basal FSH concentrations, this relation does not seem to be useful for routine pre-conceptional screening to identify women at risk for a Down syndrome pregnancy. The detection rate of Down syndrome by pre-conception basal FSH screening was only 14% at a false positive rate of 5%, whereas current first or second trimester screening tests have detection rates varying between 59 and 76%, at a false positive rate of 5% *(Wald et al., 1999)*. Incorporating pre-conceptional routine basal FSH screening into the regimen of first trimester serum screening followed by NT measurement would increase the detection rate from 85 to 87%. The relatively low detection rate and low positive likelihood ratio of basal FSH screening would result in a considerably higher number of procedure related losses of unaffected pregnancies than would maternal serum screening or NT measurement during pregnancy *(Montfrans et al., 2001)*.

In subfertile patients however, signs of depletion of the primordial follicle pool may be identified by measurements of FSH during routine subfertility evaluation. Especially in artificial reproduction technique programs, basal FSH concentrations have proven prognostic value for fecundity rates *(Muasher et al., 1988; Scott et al., 1989; Toner et al., 1991; Magarelli et al., 1996; Martin et al., 1996; Buyalos et al., 1997; Gurgan et al., 1997; Sharif et al., 1998)*.

Many clinics therefore screen for elevated basal FSH concentrations in patients undergoing assisted reproductive technology regimens. On the basis of current knowledge, women known to have elevated basal FSH concentrations, who achieve pregnancy, are likely to have an increased risk for a Down syndrome pregnancy (estimated increase 2.8-fold). These women could be informed of their increased risk. In our opinion however, non invasive screening tests such as first trimester serum screening and NT measurement should be offered first to these women, instead of chorionic villus sampling or trans-abdominal amniocentesis. Clinics offering invasive prenatal diagnostics using a risk there hold value of 1:250, could inform their patients aged >32 years of the increased risk in the presence of elevated basal FSH concentrations *(Montfrans et al., 2001)*.

Although the detection rate of basal FSH screening proved insufficient for routine screening for Down syndrome pregnancies, other markers for early depletion of the primordial follicle pool might provide a better screening test. Several other methods for measuring depletion of the primordial follicle pool are available, one of which is the clomiphene citrate challenge test, which is performed by measuring FSH concentrations before and after the administration of a fixed dosage of clomiphene citrate.

The sensitivity of the clomiphene citrate challenge test to identify women with depletion of the primordial follicle pool is reported to be higher than that of screening for elevated basal FSH concentrations (26 versus 8%) *(Barnhart & Osheroff 1998)*.

One may therefore speculate that a clomiphene citrate challenge test would have a higher sensitivity to identify women at risk for a Down syndrome pregnancy. Other authors have reported that ultrasonographic assessment of the number of antral follicles early in the follicular phase of the menstrual cycle can be used to identify women at risk for a depleted primordial follicle pool *(Scheffer et al., 1999)*.

There are however currently no data describing the relation between Down syndrome pregnancies and abnormal results of the clomiphene citrate challenge test or with a low antral follicle count *(Montfrans et al., 2001)*.

The study has several limitations, some of which may be attributed to the study design. First, the data were derived from a case–control study, which may have biased the results. For example recruitment bias may have occurred in patient and control selection, either causing overestimation or underestimation of our findings. Second, we assumed that elevated basal FSH values in women with a history of a Down syndrome pregnancy and in controls were already present before pregnancy and not due to the Down syndrome pregnancy. Although in our opinion it would be unlikely that FSH concentrations would rise specifically due to a chromosomally abnormal pregnancy, the study did not investigate basal FSH concentrations prior to pregnancy. The data would have to be confirmed in a prospective study, measuring FSH concentrations prior to pregnancy, before definitive conclusions can be drawn *(Montfrans et al., 2001)*.

8. Periconceptional intake of folate and vitamin B12 in prevention of neural tube defects and Down syndrome:

Folic acid supplementation and food fortification are associated with a significant reduction in the risk of neural tube defects (NTD) *(Ray et al., 2002)*. Genetic polymorphisms for enzymes that remethylate homocysteine to methionine, a pathway dependent on normal folate metabolism, have been associated with trisomy 21 *(Hobbs et al., 2000)* and a familial clustering of NTD and trisomy 21 has also been seen *(Barkai et al., 2003)*. Since the nondisjunction of trisomy 21 may arise either during oocyte maturation or at the time of oocyte fertilization *(Hassold & Hunt 2001)*, it is hypothesized that higher folic acid intake might

31

reduce the likelihood of such chromosomal aberrations. *Fenech et al., 1998*, most Canadian cereal grains (e.g., flour) were being fortified with folic acid, providing an additional daily average of about 0.2 mg of synthetic folic acid. This enabled studying whether food fortification was associated with a decline in the prevalence of trisomy 21 *(Ray et al., 2003)*.

Despite the limited sensitivity of maternal serum screening for detecting trisomy 21 *(Meier et al., 2002)*, this study consistently included both antenatally and postnatally detected cases, thereby reducing the risk of ascertainment bias *(Bower et al., 2001)*. Furthermore, the prevalence of trisomy 21 during the pre-fortification period was the same as in other studies *(Beaman & Goldie 2001)*. Clearly, it is difficult to detect those aneuploid pregnancies spontaneously aborted earlier than 14 week's gestation *(Ray et al., 2003)*.

We previously observed a significant and large rise in red cell folate concentrations among Ontarian women of reproductive age within 12 months of complete food fortification*(Ray et al., 2002)*, as well as a 50% decline in the prevalence of open neural tube defects*(Ray et al., 2002)*. Although 0.2 mg daily of extra synthetic folic acid may not be enough to prevent most cases of trisomy 21 cases, we would have expected some reduction, which was not so *(Ray et al., 2003)*.

These preliminary findings do not support the hypothesis that increased folic acid intake can substantially lower the population risk of fetal trisomy 21. Given the limitations of our study design, however, we believe that the hypothesis deserves further testing, including an evaluation of the interactions between maternal age, folate and homocysteine status, and the genetic polymorphisms influencing these environmental interactions *(Ray et al., 2003)*.

CHAPTER 3

PRENATAL SCREENING FOR DOWN SYNDROME

Antenatal screening for Down syndrome was first performed in the 1970's using advanced maternal age or a previous history of aneuploidy. In the 1980's, the association of Down syndrome with abnormal levels of certain specific serum markers was discovered and maternal serum screening was developed which further improved the detection rate. Screening for trisomy 21 should be offered to all women's as part of routine antenatal care. This offer should include detailed counseling about the implications and limitations of the test used in the screening program. Women should have the option as to whether they wish to have screening or not. Screening tests will not diagnose whether or not the fetus is affected by Trisomy 21, but simply place the woman in a high risk or low risk category. Being in the low risk group does not exclude the possibility of Down syndrome. Women in the high risk group should be offered diagnostic testing to establish whether or not the fetus is affected. Invasive prenatal diagnosis is associated with a risk of fetal loss of 0.5-1%. Therefore information gained from the various screening techniques (biochemical and ultrasound) is combined with maternal age to lower false positive rates and minimize unnecessary invasive testing *(Pandya 2006)*.

Over the last 10 years, new technology has improved the methods of detection of fetal abnormalities, including Down syndrome. While there are ways to diagnose Down syndrome by obtaining fetal tissue samples by amniocentesis or chorionic villus sampling, it would not be appropriate to examine every pregnancy

33

this way. Besides greatly increasing the cost of medical care, these methods do carry a slight amount of risk to the fetus *(Leshin 2007)*.

So screening tests has been developed to try to identify those pregnancies at high risk. These pregnancies are then candidates for further diagnostic testing *(Leshin 2007)*.

To improve antenatal screening services for Down syndrome, it is important to have access to data concerning the effectiveness of the screening test not only in terms of sensitivity (the detection rate) but also in terms of specificity (the false-positive rate). Improving the effectiveness of the screening test will help to reduce the harm inflicted by the screening program, particularly the anxiety experienced by women/parents in receipt of a false-positive result. However, only 54% of respondents offering serum screening for Down syndrome, either alone or in combination with nuchal translucency (NT), were able to provide data for the detection rate for serum screening and only 24% of units undertaking NT could provide information on the detection rate for this screening test *(NSC 2002)*.

The survey revealed a wide variation not only in the level of risk used as the distinction between "high risk" and "low risk", usually called the cut-off level but also in the number of weeks of gestation at which the threshold or cut-off is applied. However, the UK NSC has recently made a recommendation that for a screening test undertaken during the second trimester of pregnancy a threshold or cut-off of 1:250 at 14 weeks' gestation should be used by all maternity units. The implementation of this recommendation should decrease the variation apparent in the calculation of the risk of having a pregnancy affected by Down syndrome. In future, it will be necessary to come to an agreement about the appropriate threshold or cut-off and the number of weeks gestation at which it should be applied, for any screening test undertaken during the first trimester *(NSC 2002)*.

In the USA, 35 years of age was adopted as the screening cut-off, and pregnant women above that age were routinely offered diagnostic testing. In the UK, the age in different regions, depending on the availability of diagnostic resources *(Wald & Hackshaw 2000)*.

Another method for identifying fetuses with trisomy 21 is evaluation of the fetuses by genetic sonography and offering amniocentesis only to those patients in which the sonographic findings were abnormal. Recent studies have examined the use of second-trimester genetic sonography to identify fetuses with trisomy 21 and have reported sensitivities in women at high risk of between 60% and 91% and false-positive rates of between 5.9% and 15.8% *(DeVore et al., 1995; Bromley et al., 1997; Nyberg et al., 1998; Vintzileos et al., 1999; DeVore et al., 2000; Winter et al., 2000)*.

Ultrasound marker (nuchal translucency measurement) is associated with another two biochemical markers "pregnancy associated plasma protein-A (PAPP-A) which is decreased and free β-hCG" which is increased as screening markers in the first trimester of pregnancy. Using these three markers together with maternal age can identify 85% of affected pregnancies, with 5% false-positive rate *(Wald & Hackshaw 2000)*.

Later, several markers of Down syndrome have been discovered in maternal urine. The β-core fragment is the major metabolic product of hCG in maternal urine and second trimester levels are increased on average in Down syndrome pregnancies to a greater extent than maternal serum hCG and free-β hCG *(Cuckle 2000)*.

A very important consideration in the screening test is the age of the fetus "gestational age". The correct analysis of the different components depends on knowing the gestational age precisely. The best way to determine that is by ultrasound *(Benacerraf 1996)*.

In screening program, marker levels are described in terms of *Multiple of the Median* (MoM). This is to allow for the fact that marker levels vary with gestational age. MoM values are calculated by dividing an individual's marker level by the median level of that marker for the entire population at that gestational age in that laboratory. Using MoM values, rather than absolute levels, also allows results from different laboratories to be interpreted in a consistent *way (Leshin 2007)*.

Once the blood tests results are determined, a risk factor is calculated based on the normal blood tests for the testing laboratory. The average of normal is called the "population median". Test results are sometimes reported to doctors as *Multiples of Median* (**MoM**). The average value is therefore called 1.0 MoM *(Leshin 2007)*.

Down syndrome pregnancies have lower levels of AFP and estriol. So, their levels would be below the average and therefore less than 1.0 MoM. Likewise, hCG in Down syndrome pregnancy would be greater than 1.0 MoM. In the serum screening, the lab reports all results in either this way or as a total risk factor calculated by a software program *(Leshin 2007)*.

Basic requirement for a screening program:

There is much interest in new method of screening for Down syndrome and in many cases; such methods have been introduced into routine clinical practice before being fully evaluated *(Benn 2002)*.

Criteria for screening programs have been specified *(Cuckle & Wald 1984)*. These include a well-defined medically important disorder with known prevalence and tests that are cost-effective, safe and accessible, have well-defined performance *(Benn 2002)*.

Table (2) shows the basic requirements for a screening program that should be fulfilled by any screening procedure *(Wald et al., 2003)*.

Table (2): Basic requirements for a screening program

Aspect	Requirement
Disorder	Well defined.
Prevalence	Known.
Natural history	Medically important disorder for which there is an effective remedy available.
Financial	Cost-effective.
Facilities	Available or easily installed.
Ethical	Procedures after a screen positive result are generally agreed and acceptable both to the screening authorities and to the patients.
Test	Simple and safe.
Test Performance	Distributions of test values in affected and unaffected individuals known, extent of overlap sufficiently small, and a suitable cut-off level defined.
Access	All people who may benefit from a screening test should have access to it.

(Wald et al., 2003).

Methods of prenatal screening for Down syndrome:

These screening tests are either maternal age as the first marker, maternal serum markers, maternal urine markers and sonographic markers

Table (3): Screening tests for Down syndrome

11 - 14 weeks	▪ Nuchal translucency (NT) ▪ Combined test (NT, hCG, and PAPP-A)
14 - 20 weeks	▪ Triple test (hCG, AFP, and uE$_3$) ▪ Quadruple test (hCG, AFP, uE$_3$, and inhibin A)
11 - 14 weeks and 14 -20 weeks	▪ Integrated test (NT, PAPP-A, inhibin A, hCG, AFP, and uE$_3$) ▪ Serum integrated tests (PAPP-A, inhibin A, hCG, AFP, and uE$_3$)

(Kumar & O'brien 2004)

39

[1] Maternal age marker for Down syndrome:

In *1933, Penrose* first noted the association between Down syndrome prevalence at birth and maternal age. Numerous studies have confirmed the association using data derived from birth certificates, hospital records, cytogenetic laboratories and other sources. Prior to the introduction of biochemical screening tests, maternal age alone was used as a screening test *(Benn 2002)*.

For example, for the United States population in the 1970s, it was estimated that offering amniocenteses to all women aged 35 or more, potentially allowed 20% of Down syndrome cases to be identified *(Adams et al., 1981)*. In 1997, the detected data for the United States shows that nearly half of the Down syndrome affected pregnancies are present in women aged 35 or more *(Egan et al., 1997)*.

Researchers have established that, the likelihood reproductive cell will contain an extra copy of chromosome 21 increases dramatically as maternal ages. Therefore, an older mother is more likely than a younger mother to have a baby with Down syndrome. However, of the total population, older mothers have fewer babies; about 75% of babies with Down syndrome are born to younger women because younger women than older women have babies *(Filly 2000)*.

Only about 9% of total pregnancies occur in women 35 years or older, but about 25% of babies with Down syndrome are born to women in this age group. The incidence of Down syndrome rises with increasing maternal age as shown in **Table (4).**

Many specialists recommend that women who become pregnant at age 35 or older undergo prenatal testing for Down syndrome. The likelihood that women under 30 who become pregnant will have a baby with Down syndrome is less than 1 in 1,000 but the chance of having a baby with Down syndrome increases to 1 in 400 for women who become pregnant at age 35 *(Filly 2000)*.

The likelihood of Down syndrome continues to increase as a women ages, so that by age 49, the chance is 1 in 12. But using maternal age alone will not detect over 75% of pregnancies that will result in Down syndrome *(Filly 2000)*.

Older fathers may contribute just as much as older mothers to the dramatic increase in Down syndrome risk faced by babies born to older couples. A new study found that older fathers were responsible for up to 50% of the rise in Down syndrome risk when the mother was also over 40 *(Nazario 2003)*.

Researchers say the number of births to parents over age 35 has more than doubled in the last 20 years and this has raised questions about the role of paternal age in the risk of genetic abnormalities and birth defects *(Nazario 2003)*.

Previous studies have shown that the risk of a woman having a baby with Down syndrome rises dramatically after she reaches 35. Although this effect of maternal age on Down syndrome risk is well known, researchers say the influence of the father's age on Down syndrome has not yet been defined. Some studies have found no relationship, while other, smaller studies have suggested that older fathers may raise the risk of Down syndrome *(Nazario 2003)*.

But researchers say this study, published in *The Journal of Urology*, their findings suggest that the increase in the number of babies with the genetic abnormality born to women over 35 may be the result of a combined effect of both advanced maternal and paternal ages *(Nazario 2003)*.

The study showed that the percentage of births to women over 35 grew from 8% of all births in 1983 to 17% in 1997, and the greatest change during this period was the number of births to mothers and fathers over 40 years old, which rose by 17% and 73% respectively *(Nazario 2003)*.

Researchers found that the rate of Down syndrome among parents over 40 was 60 per 10,000 births, which is six times higher than the rate found among couples under 35 years old. Older fathers over 40 had twice the rate of Down syndrome births compared with men 24 years old and younger when they had children with women over 35 *(Nazario 2003)*.

Harry Fisch wrote that, "The paternal age has an effect on Down syndrome but only in mothers 35 years old and older. In younger women, in whom age was not a risk factor for Down syndrome, there was no paternal effect."

Among older mothers over 40, researchers found that an increase of 50% in Down syndrome risk was attributable to the advanced age of the father *(Nazario 2003)*.

In fact, researchers suggest that there is only a modest increase in Down syndrome risk for women 35-39 compared with women 30-35 years old, but the dramatic increase in Down syndrome births among women 35 to 39 years old is largely due to the influence of older fathers because older women tend to make babies with older men *(Nazario 2003)*.

Young couples preparing for family planning must be aware that advanced parental age may not only result in increasing difficulties with fertility for the parents but that children born to older parents may be at higher risk for genetic abnormalities *(Nazario 2003)*.

Table (4): Relationship of Down syndrome incidence to mother's age (Estimated rate of Down syndrome in live births by one-year maternal age)

Mothers Age	Incidence of DS	Mothers Age	Incidence of DS
Under 30	Less than 1in 1,000	40	1in 105
30	1in 900	42	1in 60
35	1in 400	44	1in 35
36	1in 300	46	1in 20
37	1in 230	48	1in 16
38	1in 180	49	1in 12
39	1in 135		

(Hook 1981)

[2] First trimester screening markers for Down syndrome:

First-trimester screening for genetic defects is now an option for pregnant women, but only if certain criteria are met, according to a new committee opinion issued today by the American College of Obstetricians and Gynecologists (ACOG). New technologies, such as measuring nuchal translucency (NT), have allowed for earlier, noninvasive screening for chromosomal abnormalities and when combined with serum screening in the first trimester, have comparable detection rates as standard second-trimester screening *(ACOG 2004)*.

First-trimester screening offers several potential advantages over second-trimester screening. When test results are negative, it may help reduce maternal anxiety earlier. If results are positive, it allows women to take advantage of first-trimester prenatal diagnosis by chorionic villus sampling (CVS) at 10-12 weeks or second-trimester amniocentesis (15 weeks). Detecting problems earlier in the pregnancy may allow women to prepare for a child with health problems. It also affords women greater privacy and less health risk if they elect to terminate the pregnancy *(Andrew & Kaunitz 2004)*.

In the past decade, research has shown an association between fetuses with certain chromosomal abnormalities and ultrasonographic findings of an abnormally increased NT (an area at the back of the fetal neck) between 10 and 14 weeks gestation. The newer first-trimester screening method includes measurement of NT, free beta subunit of human chorionic gonadotropin (ß-hCG) and pregnancy-associated plasma protein-A (PAPP-A). It has a comparable detection rate for Down syndrome as the more commonly used second-trimester screening using four serum markers (alpha-fetoprotein, ß-hCG, unconjugated estriol, inhibin-A).

44

Women who screen positive are at an increased risk for having a child with Down syndrome *(ACOG 2004)*.

Researchers developed this new method of testing because women want to know earlier in their pregnancies if there are any problems. Many women also want to avoid having an invasive diagnostic procedure such as CVS, which carries a small risk of miscarriage. However, it is important for women to recognize that a negative screen indicates that their risk of having a child with Down syndrome is reduced. This is not a diagnostic test, "said Deborah A. Driscoll *(ACOG 2004)*.

First-trimester screening can also help detect other chromosomal abnormalities such as trisomy 18. In addition, measurement of NT may help detect pregnancies at risk for major heart defects in the fetus. However, first-trimester screening cannot be used as a screening test for spina bifida *(Andrew & Kaunitz 2004)*.

According to the new ACOG Committee Opinion, sonographer training and ongoing quality assurance are essential if NT is used as a screening method. Since small differences in NT measurements can have a large impact on the risk prediction of Down syndrome, sonographers need to be monitored closely. ACOG does not recommend using the NT measurement by itself to screen for Down syndrome because it has a high positive screen rate when used without serum markers. Although first-trimester screening is an option for some women, it should only be offered if the following criteria are met:

- Appropriate ultrasound training and ongoing quality monitoring programs are in place.

- There are sufficient information and resources to provide comprehensive counseling to women regarding the different screening options and limitations of these tests.
- Access to an appropriate diagnostic test is available when screening tests are positive *(ACOG 2004)*.

Compared with second-trimester screening for chromosomal abnormalities, first-trimester screening offers couples greater privacy and earlier information. Women with positive screening results can undergo chorionic villus sampling (CVS) to confirm the results, rather than wait to undergo amniocentesis later in pregnancy -- thus affording the option of earlier, safer termination of pregnancies. However, fewer than half of the women who carried fetuses with trisomy 21 and who chose to terminate their pregnancies did so before 15 weeks' gestation. This observation suggests that limited access to both CVS and abortion might reduce the benefits associated with earlier screening. In addition, some experts express concerns regarding standard measurement of fetal-nuchal translucency *(ACOG 2004)*.

In selected centers, first-trimester screening now can be implemented. However, editorialists suggest that second-trimester screening remain the standard of care, pending results from other studies and revision of practice guidelines *(Andrew & Kaunitz 2004)*.

Table (5) show the performance of antenatal screening for Down syndrome at 10-13 weeks of pregnancy. At a 5% false positive rate, the detection rate of the combined test (based on maternal age with ultrasound and serum markers) is 13 percentage points greater than the detection rate associated with nuchal translucency measurement and maternal age alone.

Table (5): Screening performance at 10-13 weeks of pregnancy according to method (all include the use of maternal age and gestational age)

	Nuchal Translucency thickness	Nuchal Translucency +free B-HCG	Nuchal Translucency +PAPP-A	Combined test (nuchal translucency free B-HCG, PAPP-A)
FPR (%)	**DR (%)**			
1	59	62	67	72
3	68	72	77	81
5	72	77	81	85
7	76	80	84	88
9	78	82	86	90
DR (%)	**FPR (%)**			
60	1.1	0.8	0.4	0.2
70	3.8	2.4	1.4	0.8
80	10.6	7.3	4.3	2.5
90	30.9	21.5	15.0	9.7

HCG, human chorionic gonadotrophin PAPP-A, pregnancy associated plasma protein A FPR, false positive rate DR, detection rate *(Wald et al., 1999).*

Maternal serum markers for Down syndrome:

Maternal serum screening for Down syndrome is an established practice in many countries. In the second trimester human chorionic gonadotrophin (HCG) or free β-hCG is the marker of first choice, with α-fetoprotein (AFP) as the second marker and unconjugated oestriol (uE$_3$) the third *(Cuckle 2000)*.

Statistical models with parameters derived by meta-analysis predict that a three-marker combination "triple marker" will yield a 67% detection rate for a 5% false-positive rate. A fourth combination of pregnancy associated plasma protein-A, free β-hCG, AFP and uE$_3$ will yield a 70% detection rate. This is increased to 88% if ultrasound nuchal translucency is used as an additional marker *(Cuckle 2000)*.

(A) First trimester serum markers:

1. Pregnancy-Associated Plasma Protein-A marker (PAPP-A):

Pregnancy-associated plasma protein-A (PAPP-A) is a large glycoprotein tetramer produced during pregnancy by the trophoblast. Low levels of PAPP-A can also be traced in non-pregnant adults *(Brambati et al., 1993)*.

Brambati et al., 1991 first recognized the potential value of measuring maternal serum pregnancy-associated plasma protein-A (PAPP-A) in screening for fetal aneuploidy in the first trimester. Numerous studies have confirmed that

PAPP-A is low in first trimester pregnancies complicated by Down syndrome (*Wald et al., 1997*).

Maternal serum PAPP-A concentration is normally increasing rapidly during the first trimester and therefore, accurate gestational age assessment is critical. Based on maternal age and PAPP-A concentrations, an estimated 52% of Down syndrome pregnancies could be identified at the 5% false-positive rate, but this value will be dependent on the time in the first trimester that the testing is performed (*Cuckle et al., 1999*).

By 15 weeks gestation, the efficacy of this marker is lost and there is no value in performing the PAPP-A test for second trimester patients. There are data to suggest that low maternal serum PAPP-A concentrations are predictive for subsequent spontaneous abortion (*Westergaard et al., 1983*). Whether or not detecting low concentrations of PAPP-A preferentially identifies those Down syndrome pregnancies with the highest risk for fetal death is unknown (*Benn 2002*).

2. Human chorionic gonadotrophin marker (hCG):

There has been some controversy as to the value of total hCG in first trimester screening for Down syndrome. One of the studies has show good distinction between affected and unaffected pregnancies (*Haddow et al., 1998*), while others appear to show minimal utility (*Hallahan et al., 2000*).

This discrepancy appears to be explainable by differences in the gestational ages for the samples used in the various studies. Total hCG would appear to be useful for screening performed after 11 weeks gestational age, but not before that time (*Spencer et al., 2000*).

Free β-hCG is substantially elevated at 8-14 weeks gestation in Down syndrome pregnancies (*Wald et al., 1995*). It is estimated that, at the usual 5% false-positive rate, the combination of maternal age and free β-hCG measurement could result in a 42% detection rate (*Cuckle et al., 1999*). Peak concentrations of maternal serum free β-hCG normally occur at   8-10 weeks in unaffected pregnancies (*Ozturk et al., 1987*). The observation that free β-hCG is elevated in Down syndrome pregnancies at 8-10 weeks would, therefore, indicate that these anomalous concentrations cannot be attributed to a relative developmental immaturity of the affected pregnancies (*Benn 2002*).

3. Activin-A marker:

Activins are a group of homodimeric proteins consisting of two β-subunits, belonging to the family of transforming growth factor b-proteins, which are involved in cellular differentiation, proliferation and morphogenesis (*Ying 1988; Massague 1990*).

In pregnancy the placenta produces activin-A and maternal serum levels increase with gestation (*Qu & Thomas 1995*), whilst activin-B is not present in maternal serum but is present in amniotic fluid and cord serum. The development of reliable immunoassays for activins has been complicated by the fact that circulating activins may be bound to binding proteins such as follistation, but recently new assays have emerged which overcome the binding protein interferences and enable total activin-A to be measured (***Knight et al.,1996***).

4. Schwangerschafts Protein:

Schwangerschafts Protein1 (SP1) "pregnancy-specific β-glycoprotein 1" is of placental origin appearing in the maternal circulation early in pregnancy. It is also known as cancer antigen 125 (CA125). It has been investigated as a potential marker for Down syndrome in the first trimester in several studies because lower levels were reported in Down syndrome pregnancies (***Yaron & Mashiach 2001***).

The results of the different studies vary considerably. ***Brock et al.1990***, analyzed maternal serum samples from 21 Down syndrome pregnancies and 63 unaffected pregnancies matched for gestational age and length of storage. The median for SP1 level in Down syndrome pregnancies was 0.79 MoM (***Yaron & Mashiach 2001***).

Macintosh et al., 1993 examined SP1 in 692 women who underwent CVS at 6 to 12 weeks. There were 30 pregnancies with abnormal karyotypes (Down syndrome, N=14; trisomy 18=8; and eight other anomalies). The median SP1 of chromosomally abnormal group pregnancies was 0.5 MoM. Particularly for Down syndrome pregnancies, the median SP1 was 0.4 MoM. They suggested that the use of SP1 as a screening test for chromosome anomalies in the first trimester could have a detection rate of 43% for a 5% false-positive rate (***Yaron & Mashiach 2001***).

Multiple marker screening:

Most centers use two or three maternal serum markers, in addition to maternal age, in the second trimester for screening of Down syndrome but some use a fourth serum marker and increasingly centers are moving towards first trimester screening with both maternal serum and ultrasound markers (***Cuckle 2000***).

In the second trimester, the triple marker test (hCG, AFP and uE_3) has generally been adopted, but in some centers the double test (AFP and hCG combined with maternal age) is the most commonly used test. Others add the inhibin-A to the triple test to form the quadruple test (***Palomaki et al., 1995; Wald et al., 1999***).

First trimester screening for Down syndrome is performed using the maternal serum of PAPP-A, and free β-hCG associated with the ultrasound marker. **Fig. (4)** Shows the detection rate for 5% false-positive rate using maternal age and multiple marker combinations. There is considerable increase in the detection rate when multiple markers are used. About twice the number of Down syndrome pregnancies can be detected using the double test compared with screening using maternal age alone. The addition of uE_3 to AFP and total hCG increases the detection rate by about 5% if gestational age is estimated by dates, or by about 10% if it is based on an ultrasound scan (***Wald et al., 1997***).

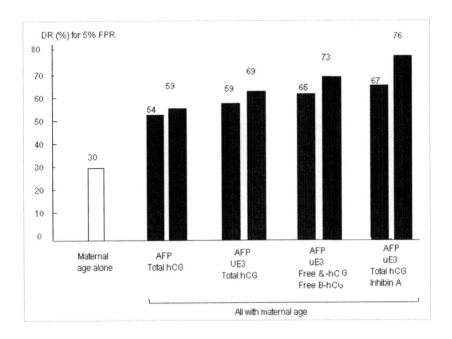

Fig. (4): Detection rate for a 5% false-positive rate according to age alone and maternal age with various combinations of markers (DR, detection rate; FPR, false positive rate; ■, gestation by dates; ■, gestation by scan) *(Wald et al., 1997)*.

Sonographic screening for Down syndrome:

Ultrasound is a noninvasive procedure that may be performed at any stage of a pregnancy (**Genetics & Public Policy Center 2007**).

The role of ultrasound in screening for Down syndrome:

Ultrasound enhances antenatal Down syndrome screening by:

- Precise gestational age of the fetus for the interpretation of serum screen results.
- Detecting major structural anomalies that occur in approximately 20% of all second-trimester Down syndrome fetuses.
- Detecting minor markers, such as nuchal fold thickness, pyelectasis, echogenic bowel, short long bones and hypoplasia of the mid-phalanx of the fifth digit, which are more commonly seen in second-trimester fetuses with Down syndrome.
- Acting in combination with serum screening in the first trimester using fetal nuchal translucency as the marker *(Egan 2002)*.

Ultrasound enhances the efficacy of either maternal age or maternal age and the serum screen for the antenatal detection of Down syndrome *(Egan 2002)*.

Assessment of fetal anatomy:

Green and Hobbins 1988, studied visualization of first trimester fetal anatomy. It was commented that the fetal limbs including elbow and knees were

54

visible by 10 weeks. The fetal face, including mandible, maxilla and orbits could be defined at 11 weeks. The ventricular system, mid-line structures, thalami, cerebellum, choroids plexus and fetal long bones and fetal digit could be well delineated by 12 weeks. The fetal hands are often open in the first trimester, making it easier to count the digit and detect the polydactyl; whereas the hand is often closed in the second trimester.

The optimal gestational age to examine the complete fetal anatomy and measure nuchal translucency is usually at 13 weeks *(Economides et al., 1999)*. There have been startling advances in the use of ultrasound for the detection of fetuses with Down syndrome. In particular, screening programs have begun using sonographic markers of Down syndrome among women at high risk for having affected fetuses. An increasing number of sonographic markers have been linked to an elevated risk of fetal Down syndrome in the second trimester and these are used for detecting fetuses at risk for Down syndrome *(Benacerraf et al., 1994; Vintzileos et al., 1997; Nyberg et al., 1998; Bahado-Singh et al., 1998)*.

As this list of sonographic markers grows the likelihood that a routine ultrasound will identify at least one marker rises dramatically. Such sonographic findings are common place in karyotypicaly normal fetuses *(Benacerraf 2000)*.

[B] First trimester ultrasound markers:

First-trimester ultrasonographic screening for trisomy 21 has gained increasing popularity since the pioneer work of *Nicolaides et al., 1992*, which first demonstrated an association between increased nuchal translucency in the first trimester and chromosomal abnormalities. Subsequent studies from the same group demonstrated that the use of nuchal translucency thickness measurement in combination with maternal age is able to detect more than 70% of affected pregnancies for a false positive rate of 5%. To further improve the detection rate of trisomy 21 in the first trimester, other ultrasonographic markers have been extensive sought *(Nicolaides 2003)*.

1. Nuchal Translucency marker:

Nuchal Scan is a sonographic prenatal screening scan to help identify higher risks of Down syndrome in fetuses, particularly for older mothers who have higher risks of such pregnancies. The scan is carried out at 11-13 weeks pregnancy and assesses the amount of fluid behind the neck of the fetus - also known as 'the nuchal translucency' **(Fig. 5)**. A large nuchal translucency has been associated with an increased risk for aneuploidy, genetic disorders, anatomic abnormalities and poor pregnancy outcomes. When obtained between 10 weeks 3 days' and 13 weeks 6 days' gestation, measurement of the NT has been shown to be a powerful sonographic marker for trisomy 21 *(Nicolaides 2006)*.

Indication:

All women, whatever their age, have a small risk of delivering a baby with a physical and/or mental handicap. The most common genetic disorder is Down syndrome with the risk rising with maternal age from 1 in 1530 pregnancies at aged 20, to 1 in 30 at aged 44 *(Nicolaides 2006)*. Whilst the only way to know for sure wheather or not the fetus has a chromosomal abnormality is by having an invasive test such as an amniocentesis or chorionic villus sampling, such tests carry an approximate 1% risk of causing a miscarriage, wheather or not the fetus is normal or affected with Down. Most women, especially those with a low risk of having a Down-affected fetus, may wish to avoid the risk to the fetus and the discomfort of invasive testing (*Nicolaides 2006*).

The aim of the nuchal scan is to estimate the risk of the fetus having Down syndrome more accurately than calculating based on maternal age alone. Only those women with significantly higher risks than that predicted for their age group, or those with an estimated risk above that of the fetal loss rate associated with amniocentesis are advised to proceed to invasive testing (*Nicolaides 2006*).

Procedure:

Nuchal scan is performed between the 11th and 13th week of gestation, because the accuracy is best in this period. The scan is obtained with the fetus in a perfect midsagittal view and a neutral position of the fetal head (neither hyperflexed nor extended, either of which can influence the nuchal translucency thickness). Carful attention should be paid to distinguish the nuchal skin from the amnion. The fetus should have a neutral neck and the image should be magnified significantly to fill 75% of the screen, and the maximum thickness is measured, from leading edge to leading edge (*Nicolaides 2006*).

Normal thickness depends on the Crown-rump length (CRL) of the fetus. Among those fetuses whose nuchal translucency exceeds the normal values, there is a relatively high risk of significant abnormality (*Nicolaides 2006*).

Accuracy:

Between 65 and 85% of trisomic fetuses will have a large nuchal thickness. Further, other, non-trisomic abnormalities may also demonstrate an enlarged nuchal transparency. This leaves the measurement of nuchal transparency as a potentially useful 1st trimester screening tool. Abnormal findings allow for early careful evaluation of chromosomes and possible structural defects on a targeted basis (*Nicolaides 2006*).

At 12 weeks of gestational age, an average nuchal thickness of 2.18 mm has been observed, however, up to 13% of chromosomally normal fetuses present with a nuchal luncency of greater than 2.5 mm, and thus for even greater accuracy of predicting risks, the outcome of the nuchal scan may be combined with the results of simultaneous maternal blood tests (*Nicolaides 2006*).

Development of nuchal translucency:

The translucent area measured (the nuchal translucency) is only usable to measure between 10 and 14 weeks' gestation, when the fetal lymphatic system is developing and the peripheral resistance of the placenta is high. After 14 weeks the lymphatic system is likely to have developed sufficiently to drain away any excess fluid, and changes to the placental circulation will result in a drop in peripheral resistance. So, after this time any abnormalities causing fluid accumulation may seem to correct themselves and can thus go undetected by making a nuchal scan (*Nicolaides 2006*).

In multiples pregnancy, NT appears to be a promising modality for screening for aneuploidy. As suggested previously, maternal serum screening in multiples has been limited because of the potential for discordance between fetuses and because of the impact of the various placentas on analytes. The NT distribution does not seem to differ significantly in singletons compared with twins. Thus, the Down syndrome detection rate in multiples should be similar to that of singletons.

Further research is still needed, but this screening modality appears to be an improvement over maternal serum screening. Some centers are already using NT measurements for screening for aneuploidy in patients with multiples and NT measurements have been used for fetus selection in patients undergoing multifetal pregnancy reduction *(Anderson 2005)*.

The study demonstrates that, in the mixed high and low-risk population, increased nuchal translucency thickness remains an extremely important first-trimester ultrasonographic marker of trisomy 21 when preformed by adequately trained operators. Among the 31 cases of trisomy 21 identified, 28 had a nuchal translucency thickness more than 95th percentile, yielding a sensitivity of 90.3% *(Souka et al., 2005)*.

Increased nuchal translucency thickness, however, had a false-positive rate for detecting trisomy 21 of 5.2%. This is not surprising, because it is well known that increased nuchal translucency is also associated with many other conditions such as congenital heart defects, genetic syndromes, and congenital structural anomalies *(Souka et al., 2005)*, in addition to other chromosomal abnormalities such as trisomy 18, trisomy 13 and Turner syndrome *(Nicolaides 2004)*.

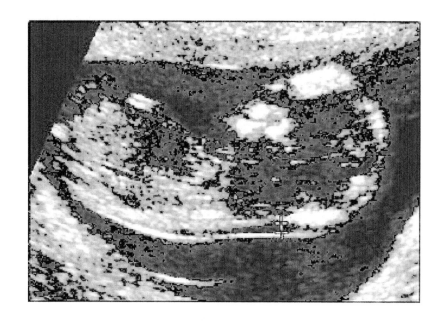

Fig. (5): Ultrasound showing fetus and NT measurement after 11-14 week *(Nicolaides 2006)*

2. Nasal bone absence:

Recently, a novel ultrasound marker, the absence of nasal bone, has been proposed as a new method to identify fetuses at risk for trisomy 21 (*Cicero et al., 2003*).

In 1866, Langdon Down noted several features in individuals with trisomy 21 which included a small nose, flat facies and poor skin elasticity. In *1997 Keeling, Hansen and Kjaer* reported an absent nasal bone in fetuses with trisomy 21. *In November, 2001, Cicero et al.,* reported in *Lancet* the association between trisomy 21 and absence of the nasal bone in fetuses with trisomy 21 examined between 11 and 14 weeks of gestation. They found that the nasal bone was absent in 72.8% of fetuses with trisomy 21, 55% with trisomy 18, and 25% with Turner syndrome. It was present in fetuses with trisomy 13, XXX, Klinefelter syndrome or triploidy. Using this marker coupled with nuchal translucency and maternal age, a risk of 1 in 300 or higher will identify 92% of fetuses with trisomy 21 with a false-positive rate of 3%. However, before one can use the presence or absence of the nasal bone as a marker for trisomy 21, the ability to identify this structure accurately is necessary (*Cicero et al., 2003*).

Identification of the Nasal Bone:

The visualization of the nasal bone was described by *Cicero et al., 2006,* For examination of the nasal bone, the image was magnified so that the head and the upper thorax only were included in the screen and a midsagittal view of the fetal profile was obtained. Because, the nasal cartilage is not a single central structure, the ultrasound transducer was parallel to the direction of the nose and the probe was gently titled from side to side to ensure proper evaluation for presence or absence of nasal bone *(Cicero et al., 2003)*.

When these criteria were satisfied, 3 distinct lines were seen at the level of the fetal nose. The first 2, which are proximal to the forehead, are horizontal and parallel to each other, resembling an "equal sign". The top line represents the skin and the bottom one, which is thicker and more echogenic than the overlying skin, represents the nasal bone. A third line, almost in continuity with the skin, but at a higher level, represents the tip of the nose *(Cicero et al., 2006)*.

The nasal bone was considered to be present when an echogenic line, thicker and more echogenic than the overlying skin, was visualized. When this third echogenic line was not visualized, or was fainter, less echogenic, and thinner than the overlying skin, the nasal bone was considered to be absent *(Sepulveda et al., 2007)*.

The Use of 2D Ultrasound to Evaluate the Nasal Bone:

Evaluation of the nasal bone was first described using 2D ultrasound in which the nasal bone was identified in the sagittal plane, which only images one nasal bone at a time. Since the nasal bone consists of two bones, to identify both bones by directing the ultrasound beam in a transverse plane. Using this approach both nasal bones can simultaneously be identified. This is a similar approach described below using 3D ultrasound *(Orlandi et al., 2005)*.

The Use of 3D Ultrasound to Evaluate the Nasal Bone:

The most important part of obtaining the image of the nasal bone is proper alignment of the beam to image this structure. To assist in the examination of the nasal bone, 3D-*multiplaner* imaging is useful because it allows the examiner to align the sagittal image of the head and accurately identify the nasal bone. The following image demonstrates the proper sagittal image for identification of the nasal bone (*Orlandi et al., 2005*).

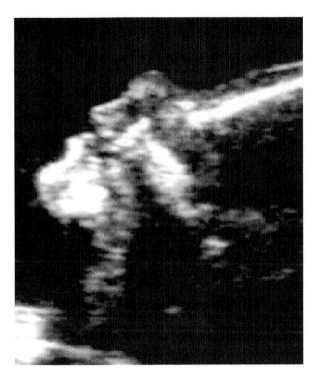

Fig. (6): An ultrasound scans for the fetal nose bone (*Otano et al., 2002*)

3. Frontomaxillary facial angle:

In fetus with trisomy 21 the frontomaxillary facial (FMF) angle, defined as the angle between the upper surface of the maxilla and the frontal bone in a mid-sagittal view of the fetal face, is substantially increased. A three-dimensional (3D) ultrasound study of 100 fetuses with trisomy 21 and 300 chromosomally normal fetuses at 11 to 13+6 weeks' gestation reported that the FMF angle was significantly bigger in the trisomy 21 than in the normal fetuses (mean 88.7°, range 75.4-104° vs. mean 78.1°, range 66.6-89.5°) *(Sonek et al., 2006)*. The FMF angle was above 85° in 69% of the trisomy 21 fetuses and in 5% of the normal fetuses. Furthermore, there was no significant association between the FMF angle and the crown-rump length (CRL) or nuchal translucency thickness. Consequently, measurement of the FMF angle is likely to be   a useful marker in addition to nuchal translucency thickness in first-trimester screening for trisomy 21 *(Plasencia et al., 2007)*.

In the measurement of the FMF angle the value of 3D ultrasonography is to ensure that the exact mid-sagittal view of the fetal face is obtained. The aims of the study were firstly, to compare the FMF angle measurement agreement and bias for a single examiner and between different examiners and secondly, to investigate the effect of deviations from the exact mid-sagittal view on the measurement of the FMF angle *(Plasencia et al., 2007)*.

Method:
The FMF angle measured using 3D volumes of the fetal face, which had been acquired from 50 chromosomally normal and 50 trisomy 21 fetuses before karyotyping by chorionic villus sampling (CVS) at 11 to 13+6 weeks' gestation.

The 3D volumes had been obtained with the fetus in the mid-sagittal plane and the transducer parallel to the long axis of the nose *(Plasencia et al., 2007)*.

All 3D examinations were carried out transabdominally with an extensive sonographer experience in first-trimester scanning and 3D ultrasound *(Plasencia et al., 2007)*.

The 3D volumes were displayed in the three orthogonal planes that compose the multiplanar mode of the 3D image. In the exact mid-sagittal plane of the fetal profile, defined by the presence of the tip of the nose anteriorly, the translucent mid-brain in the middle and the nuchal membrane posteriorly, the maxillary bone had a rectangular shape. The FMF angle a line along the upper surface of the maxilla and a line which traverses the upper corner of the anterior aspect of the maxilla extending to the external surface of the frontal bone at the point of its greatest anterior excursion were then measured *(Sonek et al., 2006)*. At 11 to 13+6 weeks of gestation the frontal bone is an echogenic line under the skin. In a previous study, it was described that in early pregnancy there is a gap between the two frontal bones which starts to close from the nasal region at around 16 weeks' gestation and moves superiorly towards the anterior fontanelle by 28 weeks *(Faro et al., 2005)*.

The transverse plane was scrolled up to obtain the standard view for measurement of the biparietal diameter (BPD). At this plane the mid-point of the BPD and occipitofrontal diameter (OFD) was determined and the head was positioned so that the midline of the OFD was at 0°. The head was then slowly rotated around the mid- point of the BPD and OFD until firstly, the tip of the nose was not visible, secondly the rectangular shape of the maxilla was altered by the superimposition of the zygomatic process of the maxilla and thirdly, the nasal bone was not visible. The angle between the original vertical line and the new OFD line at each one of the above three position was measured *(Sonek et al., 2006)*.

The FMF angle was measured at 0° and again after rotation of the head so that the OFD line formed an angle of 5°, 10° and 15° from the vertical axis. All four measurement of the FMF angle were made by the same operator, A, who on completion of the study of 50 cases repeated the measurement at 0°. The whole process was then repeated by operator B *(Plasencia et al., 2007)*.

Bland-Altman analysis was used to compare the measurement agreement and bias for a single examiner and between different examiners *(Bland & Altman 1986)*. The data were analyzed using the statistical software SPSS 12 and a P-value of less than 0.05 was considered statistically significant.

The study has utilized the multiplanar mode of 3D ultrasound to define that the sonographic markers of an exact mid-sagittal plane of the fetal face are the echogenic tip of the nose and the rectangular shape of the maxillary bone. Rotation of the head away from the vertical position of the OFD axis result in non-visibility of the tip of the nose and usually at the same angle of 4-12° the zygomatic process of the maxilla becomes visible at the anterior part of the maxilla *(Plasencia et al., 2007)*.

The data demonstrate that in the mid-sagittal plane measurement of the FMF angle is highly reproducible, and in about 95% of cases the differences between two measurements by the same observer or measurements by different observers are within 3° of each other. Although with rotation away from the mid-sagittal plane, up to at least 15°, there was a tendency for higher deviations in FMF angle, this difference was not significant in either the normal or the trisomy 21 fetuses *(Plasencia et al., 2007)*.

If the preliminary encouraging results on the difference in FMF angle between trisomy 21 and normal fetuses *(Sonek et al., 2006)* are confirmed it is likely that this measurement will be incorporated into first-trimester sonographic screening for trisomy 21. In such cases the findings of our study suggest that measurement of the FMF angle could potentially be undertaken by two-dimensional ultrasound, providd that the sonographers are appropriately trained to recognize the necessary landmarks that define the mid-sagittal plane of the face. In any case, even minor deviation from such a plane would not unduly influence the performance of the test *(Plasencia et al., 2007)*.

The increased FMF angle that observed in fetuses with trisomy 21 may be caused by a dorsal displacement of the apex of the angle (located at the front of the maxilla) with respect to the forehead. This increase can also be produced by a certain degree of frontal bossing. However, frontal bossing is not recognized as a feature of trisomy 21. The difference in the FMF angles could also result from differences in the direction of the longitudinal axis of the upper palate. A deviation of this axis toward the base of the skull would lead to an increase in the FMF angle, but this hypothesis would be difficult to test *(Snoek et al., 2007)*.

In 69 % of fetuses with trisomy 21, the FMF angle was above the 95th percentile of the normal range, and in 40% the angle was above the upper limit of the normal range. Measuring the FMF angle may also help reduce the false-positive test result rate for trisomy 21; only 2% of the affected fetuses had angle sizes below the 50th percentile. Because the FMF angle is a continuous variable,

67

likelihood ratios can be constructed for each measurement. Because no significant association exists among FMF angle, the Nuchal Translucency thickness, and the presence or absence of the nasal bone, this measurement may be included in the combined first-trimester ultrasound-based assessment of the risk for trisomy 21. Whether these results can be duplicated using 2D ultrasonography needs to be evaluated in a prospective study *(Snoek et al., 2007)*.

Measuring the FMF angle appears to be useful for screening for trisomy 21 at 11 to 13+6 weeks. However, before clinicians incorporate measurement of the FMF angle into routine screening, it is imperative that the value of the test be confirmed in prospective studies and that sonographers receive appropriate training and certification of competence in measuring the FMF angle *(Snoek et al., 2007)*.

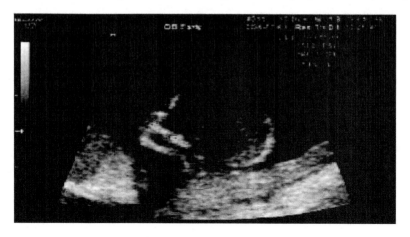

Fig. (7): The FMF angle between maxilla and frontal bones which is smaller than 90°s in a healthy fetus *(Tunç 2007)*.

Combined first -trimester screening tests:

Recent advances include using a combination of NT and biochemical markers. The combination of first trimester free β-hCG, PAPP-A, NT and maternal age is known as the Combined Test and is measured between 11 and 13 weeks. This has been reported in some studies to have a detection rate of 80-89% with a false positive rate (FPR) of 5% *(Pandya 2006)*.

Method:

The combined screen measures two analytes in the maternal serum-free beta human chorionic gonadotrophin and pregnancy-associated plasma protein A (PAPP-A). The gestational range for processing blood samples is usually between 8 and 12 weeks. It was recommended that blood is taken at 10 weeks due to the decreasing separation between affected and unaffected PAPP-A medians in Down syndrome pregnancies from 10 to 13 weeks. In practice, most bloods are taken from 10 to 12 weeks, to be assayed in the laboratory approximately 1 week before the ultrasound is performed *(Cuckle 1999)*.

Risk estimation for Down syndrome and trisomy 18 are calculated at the date of scan using multivariate probability distributions based on published methodology *(Wald et al., 1992)* and using published unaffected and affected marker means and SDs used for estimating risk of Down syndrome 21 and trisomy 18 *(Tul et al., 1999)*.

The risks are calculated for the gestation at the time of NT measurements, and thresholds are set at 1 in 300 for Down syndrome and 1 in 250 for trisomy 18.

In most cases (72%), the blood has been collected and assayed prior to the NT ultrasound, so a combined risk can be calculated immediately on receipt of ultrasound measurements.

This enables to give women the option results or receiving their results later, from the ultrasound practice or their referring practitioner. In practice, about 50% of women wait at the clinic for their result, with 22% followed within 24 hours. The remaining 28% of women have their blood taken on the day (12%), within 3 days (14%) or within 3 weeks (2%) of their NT. These results are issued within 2-3 days of receiving the blood sample. As the blood sample is usually taken prior to ultrasound, the combined screen is different from many other programs, such as the one stop clinic for assessment of risk *(Bindra et al., 2002)*.

There is a small proportion of women (<5%) who have blood collected from 13 weeks 0 days to 13 weeks 6 days, and it was concerned that there is decreased separation using the first-trimester markers between Down syndrome and normal pregnancies at 13 weeks that have been previously reported *(Malone et al., 2005)*.

The first and second trimester evaluation of risk (FASTER) study also found that the sensitivity of NT or PAPP-A alone was lowest at 13 weeks, as was overall combined test performance *(Malone et al., 2003)*.

To counteract this effect of measuring PAPP-A and NT at 13 weeks, they took into account a recommendation from a modeling report suggesting that inhibin-A, unconjugated estriol and alpha fetoprotein could also be included the standard combined screen when blood was collected at 13 weeks *(Anonymous 2000)*.

70

The report suggested that this would maximize the sensitivity for Down syndrome by increasing the sensitivity by 2.4% *(Anonymous 2000)*.

In light of this, they are trialing an approach measuring these second-trimester analytes for all pregnancies where blood was collected at 13 weeks and refer to this as the augmented screen. These pilot data do not include enough pregnancies screened by this method to validate this approach; however, they are currently monitoring all 13-week combined tests to obtain a larger sample size, which will be reported on separately *(Jaques et al., 2007)*.

Discussion:

The overall sensitivities of the combined screen for Down syndrome by the standard combined screen (88%) and the augmented combined screen (91%) are comparable to other studies which demonstrated sensitivities between 83 and 93% *(Borrell et al., 2004)*.

The difference between the combined screen group and the augmented screen group (3.2%) was small, which consistent with the modeling data (2.4% increased detection) *(Anonymous 2000)*.

The FPR was marginally greater in the standard combined screen group than in the augmented group (4.1 versus 3.9%), but there were only 760 pregnancies screened at 13 weeks, and a larger number is required to fully evaluate the augmented combined screen as a stand-alone **test** *(Jaques et al., 2007)*.

71

Using a different risk threshold of > 1 in 250, slightly lower FPRs (2.1 and 3.3%) have been demonstrated elsewhere with similar sensitivities to their cohort (91 and 88%, respectively). The sample sizes were smaller than this study at 6411 *(Wojdemann et al., 2005)* and 2860 *(Borrell et al., 2004)*, and the follow-up rate was slightly lower (96 and 97%, respectively).

Other programs, using a threshold of > 1 in 250, have demonstrated a higher FPR between 5 and 6% with varying sensitivities of 73, 82, 86 and 93%. Screening program using a risk threshold of >1 in 300 has also shown a slightly higher range of FPR, between 5.2 and 7.2% with sensitivities ranging between 83 and 92% *(Nicolaides et al., 2005)*. Overall, the 3.9% FPR in the Victorian population is extremely satisfactory and acceptable.

The method of carrying out the combined screen by genetics health uses a single central laboratory with multiple ultrasound practice, and the sensitivity of the augmented combined screen was similar to those of the one-stop method (92-93%) *(Avgidou et al., 2005)*. However, FPRs demonstrated by the one-stop method have been higher (6.8-7.5%) than those in their study. The median age of the women screened through the one-stop clinic was slightly higher at 34 years *(Avgidou et al., 2005)* than the median age of our cohort (33years), and this may have influenced the difference in FPR. At a 5% fixed FPR, the one-stop method has demonstrated a similar sensitivity for Down syndrome at 90% *(Avgidou et al., 2005)* to the population screened by genetic health (92%). As previously proposed *(Huang et al., 1997)*, these data suggest that setting a fixed FPR will produce similar sensitivities in different populations *(Jaques et al., 2007)*.

[3] Second trimester screening markers for Down syndrome:

Second trimester screening for Down syndrome is carried out between 15 and 22 weeks of pregnancy, using the double test, the triple test or the quadruple test. Either total-hCG or the free β-hCG subunit can be used in these tests, because the levels of these markers in maternal serum are highly correlated and screening performance is similar whichever one is used *(Wald & Hackshaw 2000)*.

Optimal screening requires estimation of gestational age and efficacy is maximized when results are based on an ultrasound determination of gestational age *(Wald et al., 1992; Benn et al., 1997)*. Adjustments are made to analytes concentrations to allow for some known factors that independently affect observed levels. These include maternal weight *(Neveux et al., 1996; Watt et al., 1996)*, race/ethnicity *(Watt et al., 1996; Benn et al., 1997)* and diabetic status *(Wald & Watt 1996)*.

Table (6) specifies the performance of the three second trimester screening tests (the double, triple and quadruple tests, all of which include maternal age) in two ways, showing the detection rate for specified false positive rates and the false positive rate for detection rates *(Wald et al., 1992)*.

In **Table (6)** it can be seen, for example, that at a 5% false positive rate the Down syndrome detection rates are 58%, 69% and 76%, respectively, for the double, triple and quadruple test. The quadruple test represents about a one-third increase in detection compared to the double test and about a 10% increase in detection compared to the triple test *(Wald et al., 1997)*.

73

Serum screening is, therefore, more likely to detect Down syndrome pregnancy in an older women than in a younger woman. **Table (6),** Shows the expected detection and false positive rates, for women of selected age, using triple test and a risk cut-off level of 1 in 250 (*Giacherio 2002*).

Table (6): **Maternal serum screening at 15-22 weeks of pregnancy**

	Double test (AFP, free β-HCG)	Triple test (AFP, total HCG, uE3)	Quadruple test (Triple test +inhibin-A)
FPR (%)	DR (%)		
1	32	47	54
3	49	61	69
5	58	69	76
7	65	73	80
9	69	77	83
DR (%)	FPR (%)		
60	5.5	2.7	1.6
70	9.2	5.5	3.3
80	15.9	11.1	7.0
90	29.9	24.1	16.5

AFP, alpha-fetoprotein; hCG, human chorionic gonadotrophin; uE3, unconjugated oestriol; FPR, false positive rate; DR, detection rate.
(Wald et al., 1999)

(A) Second trimester serum markers:

1. Alpha-fetoprotien marker (AFP):

AFP is included in all multiple marker screening strategies. AFP is a 70,000 MW glycoprotein produced by yolk sac and later by the fetal liver and gastrointestinal tract. It is the predominant protein in fetal circulation, present in gram/liter concentrations. Amniotic fluid contains 1/100 to 1/1000 the levels of fetal serum and maternal serum concentrations are 100 fold lower than amniotic fluid *(Giacherio 2002)*.

It is the most abundant protein in the fetal serum and may control oncotic pressure in the fetus in a manner similar to albumin postnatal. AFP is present in high concentrations in the amniotic fluid by direct fetal transmission- and in maternal serum by transplacental passage, in normal pregnancy. AFP in maternal serum normally increases through first and second trimesters *(Giacherio 2002)*.

Measurement of alpha-fetoprotin in maternal serum was carried out using a radio immunoassay *(Merkatz and Nitwosky et al., 1984)*. The discovery in early 1980s that maternal serum alpha-fetoprotien (MSAFP) levels where reduced on average in Down syndrome pregnancies brought about a radical conceptual change in antenatal screening *(Cuckle 2001)*.

The biological function of AFP in the fetus remains poorly defined *(Chard 1991)* and the reason why MSAFP levels are lower in Down syndrome pregnancies is also unclear. Studies on the synthesis of AFP by fetal liver in normal and Down syndrome fetuses have yielded inconsistent result *(Kronquist et al., 1990; Newby et al., 1997)*. High levels of AFP have been found in the placentas of affected pregnancies suggesting a defect in the secretion of AFP in the maternal circulation *(Newby et al., 1997)*.

Advanced maternal age was the main indication, and a family history of Down syndrome was another for measurement of MSAFP *(Cuckle 2001)*.

At first, a low serum AFP level was regarded as justification for prenatal diagnosis per se, regardless of the maternal age. However, it soon became obvious that the most efficient approach was to integrate all the available information by calculating an individual's risk of Down syndrome given the AFP level and maternal age *(Cuckle 2001)*.

Maternal serum AFP is detectable (~5 ng/ml) at about 10 week gestation. The co ncentration increases about 15% per week to a peak at about 25 week at approximately 180 ng/ml. The concentration in maternal serum then declines slowly until term *(Merkatz & Nitwosky et al., 1984)*. The optimal time to perform MSAFP screening is 16 weeks gestation, but it can be accurately estimated as early as 15 weeks and as late as 24 weeks. Before 14 weeks, it is of no significance *(Cuckle 2001)*.

Table (7): Conditions associated with low level of MSAFP

- **Fetal Down syndrome**
- **Trisomy 18**
- **Fetal demise**
- **Large-for-dates infants (statistical risk)**
- **Hydatiform mole**
- **Increase maternal weight**

(Graves et al., 2002)

Table (8): Conditions associated with high MSAFP levels

• **Anencephaly.**	• **Threatened abortion.**
• **Neural tube defect.**	• **Multiple pregnancies.**
• **Incorrect gestational age.**	• **Osteogenesis imperfecta.**
• **Gastrointestinal defects.**	• **Sacrococcygeal teratoma.**
- Obstruction.	• **Cystic hygroma.**
- Liver necrosis.	• **Turner syndrome.**
- Cloacal exstrophy.	• **Decrease maternal weight.**
• **Renal anomalies.**	• **Congenital skin defects.**
- Urinary obstruction.	- Abdominal wall defect.
- Poly cystic kidney.	- pilonidal cysts.
- Absent kidney.	• **Intrauterine death.**
- Congenital nephrosis.	• **Polyhydramnois.**
• **Oligohydramnios.**	

(Graves et al., 2002)

2. Human chorionic gonadotrophin (hCG):

Human chorionic gonadotrophin (hCG) is a complex glycoprotein hormone derived from syncytiotrophoblast shortly after implantation into the uterine wall. It is a heterodimer composed of two subunits (α and β) that are synthesized independently and combine before secretion. The β subunit is specific for hCG, whereas the α subunit is identical in hCG, leutinizing hormone, follicular-stimulating hormone and thyroid-stimulating hormone *(Yaron & Mashiach 2001)*. It is a placentally drived hormone, required for successful maintenance of human pregnancy *(Benn 2002)*.

Clinical application for hCG:

Bogart et al. (1987) showed that second trimester maternal serum human chorionic gonadotrophin (hCG) levels are generally higher in maternal serum when fetal Down syndrome is present. They noted that hCG appeared to be superior to MSAFP in detecting fetal chromosome abnormalities. Because of the wide-spread availability of hCG assays for pregnancy detection and monitoring, a rapid introduction of the testing as an adjunct to Down syndrome screening was possible.

Many assay techniques have been used for determining hCG involving modern techniques use immunoassays *(Cole & Kardana 1992)*. Maternal serum concentrations of intact hCG and free β-hCG show peak at weeks 9-10 and fall to a low plateau after the 20th week of pregnancy while free α-hCG does not peak until much later in pregnancy *(Braunstein et al, 1976; Ozturk et al., 1987)*. In the second trimester, assays to both α- and β-subunits will help identify Down syndrome pregnancies. However, testing with an antibody that identifies all β-subunit appears to be superior *(Wald et al., 1994)*.

It increases rapidly in the first eight weeks of gestation *(Macri et al., 1990)*. It then decreases steadily until 20 weeks, when it plateaus *(Saller & Canick 1996)*. Maternal weight and parity affect hCG levels *(Cunninghan & Williams 1997)*. An increased hCG level appears to be the most sensitive marker for detecting trisomy 21 *(Kellner et al., 1995)*. A low hCG level is associated with trisomy 18 *(Saller & Canick 1996)*. The hCG levels are normal in NTDs. By providing amniocentesis to all women older than 35 years and younger than 35 years with an age-adjusted AFP level indicating a risk of trisomy 21 equivalent to that of a 35 year old, 25 to 50 percent of cases of trisomy 21 can be detected *(Cunninghan & Williams 1997)*. The addition of hCG to the AFP screen increases detection of Down syndrome by about 40 to 50 percent over AFP alone *(Graves et al., 2002)*.

The hCG level are approximately become double in Down syndrome pregnancy. The free β-hCG becomes about 2.30 MoM *(Cuckle 2000)*.

The concentrations of hCG in maternal serum are markedly increased when fetal hydrops (generalized edema) and/or a cystic placenta is present. This is true not only for hydropic Down syndrome *(Benn et al., 2002)*, but also for Triploidy *(Benn et al., 2001)*, Turner syndrome *(Saller 1992)* and other causes of hydrops fetalies *(Saller & Canik 1996)*.

Although most cases of Down syndrome are not associated with hydrops, enlarged nuchal translucency and thickening is common and this has been

79

attributed to fluid accumulation *(Hyett et al., 1997)*. Elevated hCG may therefore be related to a disturbance in fluid homeostasis *(Chard 1991)*.

3. Unconjugated Estriol marker (uE3):

The amount of estriol in maternal serum is dependent upon a viable fetus, a properly functioning placenta and maternal well-being *(Agarwal 2003)*.

The substrate for estriol begins as dehydroepiandrosterone (DHEA) made by the fetal adrenal glands. Although present in non-pregnant patients in very low concentrations, during late pregnancy this estrogen predominates *(Tietz 1999)*. This is later hydroxylated in fetal liver and cleaved by steroid sulphatase in placenta where unconjugated fraction converts to uE3 *(Agarwal 2003)*.

Although there has been some controversy as to the value of this marker *(Macri et al., 1990)*, the cumulative data from multiple studies indicated that uE3 is nearly as useful as hCG and is more powerful than MSAFP in distinguishing between affected and unaffected pregnancies *(Wald et al., 1997)*.

Unconjugated Estriol is produced by the placenta from the fetal precursor molecule 16 alpha-hydroxydehydroepiandrosterone sulfates (DHEAS). In Down syndrome pregnancies, both uE3 and DHEAS appear to be lower than normal in the fetal liver, placental tissue, and maternal serum *(Newby et al., 2000)*. In normal pregnancies, uE3 levels increase from about 4 nmol/L at 15 weeks gestation to about 40 nmol/L at delivery. uE3 tends to be lower when trisomy 21or 18 is present and when there is adrenal hypoplasia with anencephaly *(Agarwal 2003)*.

Second-trimester maternal serum uE3 levels in Down syndrome pregnancies are approximated 75% of the values expected in normal pregnancies. Using maternal age and uE3 levels detection rate of about 45.7% at a false positive rate of 9.1 % was found *(Agarwal 2003)*.

4. Inhibin A marker:

The most promising additional marker currently available in the U.S is dimeric Inhibin A (Inh A). This glycoprotein hormone consisting of linked subunits α and βA (called inhibin-A [Inh A]) or α and βB (called inhibin-B). They are secreted from both the corpus luteum and the placenta in early pregnancy, whereas after 12 weeks the placenta becomes the major source of inhibin. They suppress the secretion of follicle stimulating hormone by the pituitary gland but their function during pregnancy has not been established *(Wald & Hackshaw 2000)*.

Maternal serum Inh A levels remain almost constant during gestational weeks 15 to 20. In several studies, Inh A levels in all Down syndrome cases are greater than the median for normals, and average approximately 2 MoMs. In retrospective analyses, the addition of Inh A to the Triple Test markers improved the detection rate for Down syndrome by 4 to 10%, up to approximately 75%, while maintaining   a fixed false positive rate of 5%. Alternatively, it is possibly to use cutoffs that will maintain detection rates of 65-69%, but reduce the false positive rate by 2% *(Giacherio 2002)*.

Currently, Inh A assays are only available in a microtiter plate ELISA format, which can be labor intense and expensive to perform for many laboratories. Short term prospects for the automation of Inh A assays, similar to that which

81

already exists for AFP and hCG, do not appear promising. Most instrument vendors appear to be cautiously biding time on the issue, waiting for further evidence of its ultimate utility. The growing research interest in using first trimester maternal serum markers such as pregnancy associated plasma protein A (PAPP-A) and free beta subunit of hCG in conjunction with more sensitive ultrasound parameters to predict risk will likely also serve to discourage automation of Inh A assays *(Giacherio 2002)*.

In the absence of any national policy or recommendation on multiple marker screening, each institution may have to examine its program to decide which approach best suits their needs *(Giacherio 2002)*.

There is a moderately strong correlation between the maternal serum concentrations of hCG and Inh A in both affected and unaffected pregnancies *(Wald et al., 1996)*. Nevertheless, Inh A still provides good distinction between affected and unaffected pregnancies alone or in combination with other tests and this can include hCG *(Benn 2002)*.

5. Lens culinaris agglutinin reactive AFP (AFP-L3):

Recently, there was found that AFP-L3 was significantly higher in women who were pregnant with a fetus with Down syndrome and that AFP-L3 could be a useful biochemical marker for prenatal Down syndrome screening *(Yamamoto et al., 2001)*. AFP-L3 is a variant of AFP *(Azuma et al., 2002)*.

This variant can be determined by electrophoresis. In contrast to the low levels of maternal serum AFP that are associated with Down syndrome, maternal serum AFP-L3 levels were significantly higher in cases of Down syndrome than among the unaffected pregnancies. In normal pregnancy, it is known that AFP-L3 gradually decreases as pregnancy progresses *(Taketa 1995)*. This is considered to be a reflection of fetal liver maturation. It was previously noted that a high level of AFP-L3 was detected in the liver tissue of fetuses with Down syndrome *(Yamamoto et al., 2001)*. Therefore, it is assumed that a high level of AFP-L3 in Down syndrome cases reflects immaturity of the fetal liver *(Azuma et al., 2002)*.

It is well known that AFP is a glycoprotein produced by the fetal liver, hepatocellular carcinoma and yolk sac tumours. The carbohydrate structure of human AFP has been analysed using preparations purified from ascites fluid of a patient with hepatocellular carcinoma *(Yoshima et al., 1980)* and a yolk sac tumour *(Yamashita et al., 1983)*. The sugar chain microheterogeneities of AFP, especially *Lens culinaris* agglutinin-reactive AFP (AFP-L3), have been studied using lectin affinity electrophoresis in relation to hepatocellular carcinoma *(Breborowicz et al., 1981; Taketa et al., 1993; Yamashita et al., 1996)*. The relationship between AFP glycoforms in maternal serum at the second trimester and Down syndrome affected pregnancies has only been determined using Concanavalin A *(Gembruch, 1987; Kim, 1990; Los et al., 1995)*. In this study, we determined the percentage of AFP variants that react with lectins as a way to find out whether the analysis of the carbohydrate chain microheterogeneities of maternal serum AFP could be useful for prenatal Down syndrome screening *(Yamamoto et al., 2001)*.

Triple marker test:

A large prospective study reported that the combination of hCG, AFP and uE_3 as markers for Down syndrome eventually resulted in the triple test.

Subsequent to this study, triple marker serum screening was incorporated into clinical practice (*Haddow et al., 1992*).

In the second trimester, AFP and uE_3, two of the markers of the triple test increase with gestational age, while hCG, the third marker decreases. Expressed in MoM values, maternal serum AFP and uE_3 are on average, reduced by approximately 25% in pregnancies with Down syndrome and levels of hCG are approximately double (*Wald & Kennaed 1992*).

Fig. (7) shows the distribution of the three markers at 15- 22 weeks of pregnancy. The most effective way to use the information on maternal age and the three serum markers is to estimate the risk of having an affected pregnancy. The triple test is a screening test "identification of an increased risk" and not a diagnostic test. The triple marker test is able to identify women whose risk of carrying a child with Down syndrome is equal to or greater than the risk of women of 35 years of age or older (*Ormond et al., 1996*).

When the risk exceeds the cut-off level (1 in 250), invasive testing in the form of amniocentesis is offered (*Mueller & Young 1998*).

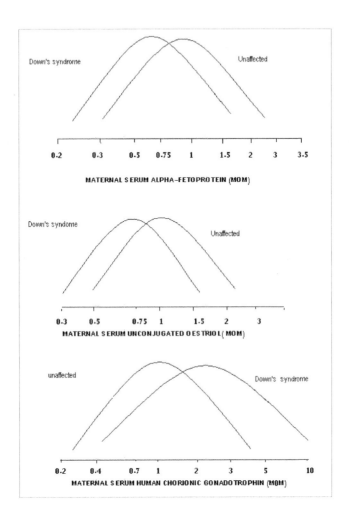

Fig. (8): Gaussian relative frequency distributions of maternal AFP, uE3, and hCG in pregnancies with Down syndrome and in unaffected pregnancies at 15-20 weeks gestation *(Wald et al., 1994)*.

When the test is performed, it is important to know the gestational age of the unborn baby, the age of the mother, her weight and her ethnicity, whether she is diabetic and whether it is a twin pregnancy. If any one of these factors is reported inaccurately, a false positive or false negative result may occur (*Benn et al., 2001*).

The Triple Test is currently the most widely utilized prenatal screening tool for the detection of Down syndrome. It utilizes maternal serum levels of a fetal marker (AFP), a placental marker (hCG) and a fetal-placental unit function marker (uE3). By measuring maternal serum levels of these markers in the 15th through 20th gestational week and following up screen positive cases with amniocentesis, 80% of neural tube defects and 65-69% of Down syndrome cases can be detected. A normal screen result reduces the likelihood of having a Down syndrome baby, but does not exclude it (*Giacherio 2002*).

Perhaps the major concern with the Triple Test and the source of much confusion with patients is the false positive rate of the test. In order to achieve the relatively high detection rate for Down syndrome, the cutoffs for the screening tests are set so that 5 to 7% of normal pregnancies will have an abnormal Triple screen result. If one assumes an overall population incidence of 1 in 1000 for Down syndrome, at a false positive rate of 6% the test will call 60 normal pregnancies abnormal for every one case of Down syndrome detected. Because the computer algorithm uses the marker MoMs to modify the age specific risk, screening a higher incidence population such as women over the age of 35 will produce a higher detection rate of Down Syndrome (approximately 80%) but also a higher false positive rate (up to 25%) (*Giacherio 2002*).

Because of the high costs and risks of amniocentesis and the anxiety produced by a screen positive result, much emphasis has been placed on additional testing to either reduce the false positive rate, increase the detection rate for Down Syndrome or both *(Giacherio 2002)*.

In retrospective analyses, the addition of Inh A to the Triple Test markers improved the detection rate for Down Syndrome by 4 to 10%, up to approximately 75%, while maintaining a fixed false positive rate of 5%. Alternatively, it is possible to use cutoffs that will maintain detection rates of 65-69%, but reduce the false positive rate by 2% *(Giacherio 2002)*.

The quadruple test:

Adding the measurement of inhibin-A to the triple test comprises the quadruple test. The quadruple test represents about a one-third increase in detection compared to the double test (AFP and HCG) and about a 10% increase in detection compared to the triple test. The extra cost of adding one or two serum markers to the double test is relatively small in relation to the improved efficacy. It has been concluded that the quadruple test is the second trimester screening test of choice *(Wald et al., 1997)*.

Table (9): The detection rates of Down syndrome using the triple test at risk of, 1 in 250 at different maternal ages

Maternal age	Detection rate (%)	False-positive rate (%)
25	36	3
03	45	5
35	66	13
40	89	41
45	99	79

(Kennard & Wald 1995)

(B) Second-Trimester Ultrasound Aneuploidy Markers:

Thirty percent of fetuses with trisomy 21 have a major structural malformation. Congenital cardiac anomalies are the commonest (up to 40%) and of these atrioventricular canal defects and ventricular septal defects are the most frequent (*Pandya 2006*).

Trisomy 21 in the second trimester is also associated with nasal bone hypoplasia, increased nuchal fold thickness, duodenal atresia, echogenic bowel, mild hydronephrosis, shortening of the femur or humerus, sandal gap and clinodactyly or midphalanx hypoplasia of the fifth finger. If the second trimester scan demonstrates major defects, it is advisable to offer fetal karyotyping, even if these defects are apparently isolated (*Pandya 2006*).

The prevalence of such defects is low and therefore the cost implications are small. If the defects are either lethal or associated with severe handicap, such as hydrops or duodenal atresia, fetal karyotyping constitutes one of a series of investigations to determine the possible cause and thus the risk of recurrence (*Pandya 2006*).

Minor fetal defects or soft markers are common and not usually associated with any handicap unless there is an underlying chromosome abnormality (*Vintzileos et al., 1997*).

Routine karyotyping of all pregnancies with these markers, therefore, would have major implications, both in terms of miscarriage and financial cost. In this situation, it is best to base counseling on an individual estimated risk for chromosomal abnormality (**Pandya 2006**).

The overall risk for chromosomal abnormalities increases with the total number of defects identified. It is therefore recommended that when a defect/marker is detected, a thorough ultrasound examination is done for other features of the chromosomal abnormality known to be associated with that defect, because the presence of additional defects increases the risk substantially (**Pandya 2006**).

One promising marker for Down syndrome, which was recently described, is nasal bone hypoplasia. This is defined as a nasal bone that is not visible or has a length of less than the 3rd centile for gestational age in the second trimester. One study examined 1046 pregnancies undergoing amniocentesis for fetal karyotyping at 15-22 weeks gestation (**Cicero et al., 2003**). The nasal bone was hypoplastic in 62% of fetuses with trisomy 21, but in only 1% of chromosomally normal fetuses. Nasal bone hypoplasia was commoner in normal Afro-Caribbean fetuses (8.8%) than in normal Caucasian fetuses (0.5%). Although much more evidence needs to be gathered, it seems likely that this marker will have a major impact on Down syndrome screening and should be incorporated into the detailed second trimester anomaly scan (**Pandya 2006**).

The estimated risk can be derived by multiplying a priori maternal age related risk by the likelihood ratio of the specific defect. The best has estimates of both the positive and negative likelihood ratios for each of the common markers of trisomy 21. On the basis of these data the likelihood ratio for trisomy 21 if there is no detectable defect or marker is 0.30. In each case the likelihood ratio is derived by dividing the incidence of a given marker in trisomy 21 pregnancies by its incidence in chromosomally normal pregnancies. For example, an intracardiac echogenic focus is found in 28.2% of trisomy 21 fetuses and in 4.4% chromosomally normal fetuses, resulting in a positive likelihood ratio of 6.41 (28.2/4.4) and a negative likelihood ratio of 0.75 (71.8/95.6) (*Pandya 2006*).

Consequently, the finding of an echogenic focus increases the background risk by a factor of 6.41, but at the same time absence of this marker reduces the risk by 25%. Thus, in a 25 year old woman undergoing an ultrasound scan at 20 weeks of gestation, the a priori risk is around 1 in 1000. If the scan demonstrates an intracardiac echogenic focus, but the nuchal fold is not increased, the humerus and femur are not short and there is no hydronephrosis, hyperechogenic bowel or major defect, the combined likelihood ratio should be 1.1 (6.41 x 0.67 x 0.68 x 0.62 x 0.85 x 0.87 x 0.79) and consequently her risk remains at around   1 in 1,000 (*Pandya 2006*).

The minor markers:

The minor markers are findings, which are commonly seen among normal fetuses, although they have a higher frequency in fetuses with aneuploidy (*Nyberg et al., 1998*).

Individuals with Down syndrome have slightly shorter long bones compared to normal, not only in infancy and childhood but also in pathologic evaluations of second trimester fetal specimens (*Simmons et al., 1989*).

Although it is well accepted that fetuses with Down syndrome have slightly short humeri and femora, the degree of shortening is very mild and overlaps

91

extensively with the normal range (*Lockwood et al., 1987; Benacerraf et al., 1987; Nyberg et al., 1990*).

Because the different bone dimensions in fetuses of different racial and ethnic backgrounds may also have an impact on this measurement, there is a wide variation in the use of this marker among different practitioners. In clinical use, slight shortenings of the femur and the humerus convey likelihood ratios of 2.2 and 2.5 times the age-based risk for Down syndrome, respectively (*Nyberg et al., 1998*).

Fetal pyelectasis, also a minor marker for Down syndrome, is common among normal fetuses. There is an increased incidence of pyelectasis in fetuses with Down syndrome compared with the normal population, with 20-25% of fetuses with Down syndrome having dilatation of the renal pelvis (*Benacerraf et al., 1990*).

Hyperechoeic bowl was first shown to be a sonographic marker for Down syndrome in 1993 (*Nyberg et al., 1993*). It is present in approximately 12.5% of second-trimester fetuses with Down syndrome. Despite this low sensitivity, the specificity is high since the incidence of hyperechoic bowel in the general population is only 0.6% (*Bromley et al., 1994*).

Small calcifications in the papillary muscle particularly in the left ventricle are commonly seen in second-trimester fetuses and are present in approximately 5-10% of normal fetuses (*Bromley et al., 1995; Shipp et al., 2000*).

An association between those findings and chromosomal abnormalities was demonstrated in 1995 (*Brown et al., 1994; Lehman et al., 1995*). On subsequent studies, they found that 18% of fetuses with Down syndrome and 5% of normal fetuses displayed these sonographic markers *(Bromley et al., 1995)*.

There are other characteristic fetal Down syndrome sonographic markers that are even more difficult to use clinically than those described above. These include hypoplasia of the middle phalanx of the fifth digit, separation of the great toe (sandal-gap foot), slight heart rate disorders, fetal ear measurement abnormalities and others *(Benacerraf et al., 1990; Gill et al., 1994; Shipp et al., 1997; Shimizu et al., 1997)*.

In summary, the second-trimester ultrsonographer may act as a prenatal dysmorphologist looking for major or minor markers that have been associated with fetal Down syndrome. If the markers are present, the risk for fetal Down syndrome is increased; if they are absent, the risk is decreased *(Vintzileos & Egan 1995)*.

[4] Urinary markers:

Several biochemical markers of Down syndrome in maternal urine were first investigated during the 1990s, including total oestriol, hCG and the most promising marker, urinary β-core hCG *(Wald et al., 1997)*.

The urinary screening test would have the advantage of being easy to collect, pain free and not requiring that the women present at a specialized center for the screening to be performed. Urine sample does not require centrifugation and separation of fluids. The risk of serum born infections is minimized in urine testing *(Cole et al., 1999)*.

93

Both maternal serum intact hCG and free-β subunit are elevated in Down syndrome pregnancies, but the extent of elevation is greater for free β-hCG (**Wald et al., 1993**).

It has been suggested that the hCG molecule is less stable in affected pregnancies. The major metabolic product, β-core hCG, is excreted in urine. This in turn led to the hypothesis that breakdown products of the β-subunit of hCG excreted into the urine may be more elevated than the circulating molecules (***Cuckle et al., 1994***).

The β-core fragment is the major metabolic product of hCG in maternal urine and second trimester levels are increased on average in Down syndrome pregnancies to greater extent than maternal serum hCG and free-β hCG (***Cuckle 2000***).

Later, a multicentre study of 6730 women (including 39 with affected pregnancies) confirmed that urinary β-core hCG is raised in Down syndrome pregnancies (70% higher than unaffected pregnancies) but the large overlap in distributions of affected and unaffected pregnancies means that it is unlikely to be useful marker in screening (***Cuckle 1999***).

Urine is safer medium than blood and may be more acceptable to women since not only is venepuncture avoided but also the test can be performed without seeing a doctor (***Cuckle 2000***).

Although this does not mean that urinary β-core hCG can replace the maternal serum hCG assays for Down syndrome screening. **Firstly**, the standard deviation of the urine marker is very wide, partly because only a random urine sample is available and the result is similar to serum free β-hCG. **Secondly,** there is significant heterogeneity between the published studies, so the overall average value may be misleading. This is possibly due to differences in assay method, study design and the integrity of urine samples during transport and storage *(Cuckle 2000).*

Other urinary hCG species –free-β hCG and hyperglycosylated hCG –are elevated on average in affected pregnancies although fewer cases have been tested than for β-core hCG. In contrast maternal urine total estrogen and total oestriol levels are reduced on average in Down syndrome pregnancies. None of the urinary markers perform well in the first trimester of pregnancy *(Cuckle 2000).*

The 3-D ultrasound and prenatal diagnosis:

Three-dimensional or volume ultrasonography acquires a volume (rather than slice) of ultrasonographic data which is then stored. This stored data can be reformatted and analyzed in numerous ways. For example, surface rendering involves projecting the surface of a structure on to the screen, which allows curved structures, such as the fetal face, to be viewed in a single image that appears photographic in nature. The difference between 3-D and 4-D ultrasound is that in 4-D ultrasound the three-dimensional view can be seen in real time. In both, substantial post-processing rendering is required to get the image detail and benefits of the technique *(Benacerraf et al., 2006).*

Suggested advantages of three-dimensional ultrasound compared to two-dimensional ultrasound in obstetrics include the following:

- Three-dimensional ultrasound appears to be less operator dependent and provides a superior display of structures with complex anatomy compared to conventional ultrasonography.

- Orientations and planes not available with two-dimensional ultrasound, because of anatomic constraints or fetal portion are available with three-dimensional ultrasound.

- Volume date may be reviewed millimeter by millimeter after acquisition, simulating real-time scanning.

- Archived volume data with suspected fetal anomalies may be reviewed with other physicians after the patient has left the department and data may be transmitted via the internet to other locations.

- Three-dimensional ultrasound has improved accuracy of volume measurements to measure regular and irregular objects.

- Volume-rendered images are easily recognizable by both parents and physicians, which may facilitate decisions by families regarding continuing or terminating the pregnancy and are also said to enable patients to bond more effectively with the fetus. It may also assist them with making lifestyle changes, such as stopping smoking or excessive alcohol intake (*Benacerraf et al., 2006*).

Limitations of three-dimensional ultrasound are as follows:

- Suboptimal volume-rendered images are obtained if there are inadequate amniotic fluids surrounding the structure of interest. This is a major limitation with oligohydramnios and as the fetus progresses towards term. The adjacent structures cannot be excluded from the rendered volume in these cases and this interferes with surface rendering.

- Unacceptable surface rendering occurs with unfavorable fetal position and with adjacent or superimposed structures (e.g., limbs).

- Image processing of the volume data may take additional time on the part of the examiner.

- Real-time capacity is not generally available with three-dimensional ultrasound. (Real time three-dimensional ultrasound is also known as 4-D ultrasound.) Whereas 3-D ultrasound is a static display of the various reformatting techniques based on the acquisition of a static volume, 4-D ultrasound displays a continuously updated and newly acquired volume in any rendering modality creating the impression of a moving structure. The time vector (the fourth dimension) makes it possible to perceive a rapid update of the successive individual images displayed on the monitor at very short intervals which creates the impression of a real time measurement, and enables the user to see fetal motion in almost real-time (***Benacerraf et al., 2006***).

[5] Combined use of both biochemical and ultrasonographic   markers:

An ultrasound examination is commonly performed for patients with maternal serum screen-positive results. This ultrasound minimally may be used to correct a major error in gestational age that may have been sufficient to explain the screen- positive result. Second trimester ultrasound may identify specific anatomic anomalies and/or markers that have been associated with Down syndrome (*Drugan et al., 2000; Smith-Bindman et al., 2001*).

Modification of risk using ultrasound-derived likelihood ratios that reflect the presence or absence of specific markers needs to be approached cautiously. In Down syndrome fetuses, the presence of more than one marker occurs more often than expected by chance and therefore, likelihood ratios for each marker cannot be treated as independent factors (*Nyberg et al., 2001*).

Additionally, biochemical tests and ultrasound findings are not necessarily independent *(Souter et al., 2002)*. In their meta-analysis, **Smith-Bindman et al., 2001** concluded that none of these ultrasound markers alone is sufficient to be clinically useful.

Wald et al., 1997 have expressed the opinion that modifying a positive second trimester maternal serum screening result by ultrasound should be avoided because true-positive will be missed. However, the policy also needs to be viewed in the context of the choice of cut-off selected for serum screening and the fact that an ultrasound examination will be an integral component of the management of screen-positive patients. Use of ultrasound data to modify risk might, with an appropriate risk cut-off, resulting in a substantial reduction in the number of amniocenteses performed with only a small reduction in the detection rate *(Egan et al., 2001)*.

Recently, a protocol that combined the quadruple test with nuchal thickness and long bone measurement was developed. This provisional study indicated combined second trimester screening might achieve an approximately 90% detection rate at the 5% false-positive standard *(Kaminsky et al., 2001)*.

In the first trimester, maternal serum analytes can be combined with each other or with the ultrasound markers to produce highly effective screening protocols. Interpretation of first trimester biochemical tests should be based on an ultrasound measurement of gestational age because the serum analytes concentrations are highly gestational age-dependent. Because of the superior discriminacy power of NT and the need for first trimester ultrasound to accurately assess gestational age, the serum test have, thus far, been largely viewed as adjunctive to ultrasound screening *(Benn 2002)*.

Integrated test:

The Integrated Test is the most recent screening test for Down syndrome *(Wald et al., 2003)*. The integrated test is done in two parts:

- The first part is done during the first trimester, and includes an ultrasound examination of the fetus to measure nuchal translucency and a test from the mother's blood to measure PAPP-A.
- The second part is done at 15 to 20 weeks of gestation, which tests the mother's blood level of alpha-fetoprotein, unconjugated estriol, hCG, and inhibin A *(Canick et al., 2008)*.

The performance of this test is reported to be better than that of all others. The model of screening described by *Wald & Hackshaw 1997* has the major theoretical advantage of a high detection rate (DR) of 94% for a FPR of 5% or alternatively 85% DR with a 1% FPR *(Wald et al., 2003)*.

The SURUSS trial found that for a fixed DR of 85% the FPR for the integrated test was 1.2%. However, the data available at present is from a single

99

retrospective study and large prospective trials are currently being conducted *(Wald et al., 2003)*.

The integrated test requires two stage screening and a proportion of women may fail to attend for the second stage test. In addition, for women who complete the test, the result is not obtained until after   16 weeks. Termination of pregnancy is more traumatic at this stage since it usually requires a medical abortion rather than surgical, and the mother may have already felt the fetal movements. The same argument could of course be applied to the second trimester anomaly scan at 18 to 23 weeks *(Pandya 2006)*.

Although the combined test may have a lower DR than the integrated test, it does yield a result in the first trimester, thus allowing an early surgical (or medical) termination, which may be less traumatic for the mother *(Pandya 2006)*.

Integrating first and second trimester screening:

The term "integrated screening" has been applied to the situation in which Down syndrome tests are performed in both the first and second trimesters but risk is only presented to patients after the completion of the second trimester component *(Wald et al., 1999)*.

The integrated test takes advantage of the fact that different screening markers discriminate between the presence and absence of Down syndrome at different times in pregnancy *(Wald et al., 1999)*.

Through the 1990s there was a steady increase in extent and complexity of Down syndrome screening. Six maternal serum markers became generally available: AFP, total hCG, free β-hCG, PAPP-A, inhibin-A, and uE_3. Three serum markers (free β-hCG, uE_3 and AFP) were shown to be effective both in first and second trimesters blood samples *(Cuckle 2001)*.

Several ultrasound markers were investigated and nuchal translucency (NT) emerged as the single most powerful marker, although it was only effective in the first trimester *(Cuckle 2001)*. Simultaneously using markers from both first and second trimesters yields a better screening performance than using markers in either trimester alone *(Wald et al., 1997)*. The effect is large because first trimester nuchal translucency measurement and PAPP-A levels are practically uncorrelated with the second trimester serum markers *(Wald et al., 1996; Lambet-Messerlain et al., 1998; De Basio et al., 1999)*.

The use of a first and second trimester integrated test represents a departure from current screening practice in that information is being used from tests performed over different periods of the pregnancy and held until all the information is to hand. The information is then appropriately combined to provide the woman with a single screening risk estimate result *(Wald & Hackshaw 2000)*.

This approach yields a detection rate that is higher than any other test at a given false positive rate. Indeed the performance of such screening is so high that it becomes more appropriate to examine the performance by comparing false positive rates at specified detection rates, because at high detection rates of around 80% and 90% the percentage scale, with its maximum of 100%, tends to conceal improvements in performance *(Wald & Hackshaw 2000)*.

101

For example, using the integrated test at a 5% false positive rate, the detection rate is 94% compared with 85% using the first trimester-combined test alone. The improvements of nine percentage points in the detection rate dose not appear large. However, at a fixed 85% detection rate, the first trimester combined test would be associated with a 5% false positive rate while the integrated test has only a 1% false rate, representing an 80% reduction in the number of false positives for the same number of Down syndrome pregnancy detected. This leads to a corresponding reduction in the number of amniocenteses required. Amniocentesis is associated with a 0.9% rate of fetal loss *(Wald et al., 1997)*.

Such a large reduction has an important impact on the safety of screening because it means that many amniocenteses performed on women with unaffected pregnancies can be avoided without reducing the number of Down syndrome pregnancies detected *(Wald & Hackshaw 2000)*.

Table (10) shows the performance of the integrated test and its variants compared with the best first and second trimester tests, by giving the false positive rates corresponding to specified detection rates, and the odds of being affected given a positive result (OAPR). The OAPR is mainly influenced by changes in the false positive rate rather than changes in detection rate. For example, an 85% detection rate can be achieved with an OAPR of 1:7, significantly more favorable than with the second trimester quadruple test (1:77) or the first trimester combined test (1:35) *(Wald & Hackshaw 2000)*.

Table (10): Performance of integrated screening and comparison with the best screening tests in the first and second trimesters

Integrated screening						
	Full integrated test	Without PAPP-A	Without inhibin-A	Without NT	second trimester quadruple test†	first trimester combined test‡
DR (%)	FPR (%)					
0.1	0.1	0.1	0.2	1.4	3.3	0.8
0.2	0.2	0.2	0.4	2.2	4.8	1.4
0.4	0.4	0.4	0.7	3.4	7	2.5
1	1	1	1.5	5.5	10.5	4.8
2.2	2.2	2.2	3.4	9.4	16.5	9.7
Odds of being affected given a positive result						
70	1:1	1:1	1:2	1:12	1:29	1:7
75	1:2	1:4	1:3	1:18	1:40	1:11
80	1:4	1:8	1:6	1:26	1:55	1:20
85	1:7	1:15	1:11	1:40	1:77	1:35
90	1:15	1:31	1:24	1:65	1:114	1:67

*First trimester nuchal translucency measurement, pregnancy associated plasma protein A (PAPP-A) plus second trimester quadruple test.

†AFP, uE3, total hCG and inhibin - A.

‡Nuchal translucency, PAPP-A, freeB –HCG.

(Wald et al., 1999)

Provided nuchal translucency measurement is retained as part of the integrated test, integrated screening has a substantially better screening performance than either the second trimester quadruple test or the first trimester combined test. If ultrasound facilities are not sufficiently developed for reliable nuchal translucency measurements, the integrated test without nuchal translucency can be used. This still has a performance that is better than the second trimester quadruple test *(Wald &Hackshaw 2000)*.

Some screening units may wish to measure free β-hCG or total hCG in the first trimester instead of the second trimester. **Table (11)** shows the screening performance of these variants with and without nuchal translucency measurement. They are reasonable alternatives to the standard approach *(Wald & Hackshaw 2000)*.

Table (11): Performance of variants of the integrated test: comparison of total and free β-hCG in the first trimester with and without nuchal translucency measurement.

Integrated screening using first trimester:				
	NT, PAPP-A, total hCG	PAPP-A, total hCG	NT, PAPP-A, free β-hCG	PAPP-A, free β-hCG
FPR (%)	DR(%)			
1	83	61	85	65
3	90	75	91	78
5	93	81	94	84
DR (%)	FPR (%)			
70	0.2	2.0	0.1	1.5
30	0.6	4.4	0.5	3.4
90	2.9	11.4	2.3	9.3
First trimester NT, PAPP-A, and either free β- hCG or total hCG and second trimester AFP, uE3 and inhibin-A				

(Wald et al., 1999).

First versus second trimester screening:

Second and first trimester screening for Down syndrome were initially seen as competitive and arguments were put forward as to why one might be better than the other.

First, arguments in favor of second trimester screening included the fact that it was established and accepted. **Second,** the screening performance was good (76% detection rate for a 5% false positive rate using the quadruple test). **Third,** AFP measurement in the second trimester permitted screening for neural tube defects (anencephaly and spina bifida), which is not possible with first trimester screening.

Lastly, the diagnostic test available, amniocentesis, was generally judged to be a simple procedure to perform. Some also regarded it as being slightly safer than chorionic villus sampling (CVS), but the evidence on this is not firm *(Wald et al., 1997)*.

The main advantage of first trimester screening is that it permits an earlier diagnosis and therefore an earlier termination of pregnancy if an affected pregnancy is diagnosed. In some countries, such as the UK, this can mean that a different method of termination may be carried out *(Wald & Hackshaw 2000)*.

The method that tends to be offered earlier in pregnancy, suction curettage, is widely regarded as less distressing and possibly safer than the later method of prostaglandin induction. On the other hand, some countries perform suction curettage as a method of termination even at 16-18 weeks of pregnancy so the termination issue with respect to safety may be more a matter of local professional for any differences in the practice than whether one method of screening is more appropriate for any particular period of pregnancy *(Wald & Hackshaw 2000)*.

In first trimester screening some affected pregnancies will be identified that would have naturally terminated few weeks later. Some would argue that first trimester screening represents an unnecessary intervention and may cause pointless grieving. Others have argued that an elective termination of a pregnancy destined to miscarry is less distressing than the natural event *(Wald & Hackshaw 2000)*.

However, the debate over the pros and the cons of first and second trimester screening is unnecessary, since by integrating screening information obtained in the first and second trimester, a screening test is made available that is far more effective than any previously described. This test is called the integrated test *(Wald & Hackshaw 2000)*.

First Trimester Screening Advantages if results are negative, it may help reduce the mother's anxiety earlier in the pregnancy — however, and it is not a diagnostic test. A negative screen only indicates that the risk of having a child with Down syndrome is reduced.

If results are positive, prenatal diagnosis can be performed in the first trimester by chorionic villus sampling (CVS) at 10 to 12 weeks, or by an amniocentesis in the second trimester (after 15 weeks) to determine if the fetus is affected.

Determining problems earlier in the pregnancy allows women to prepare for a child with health problems. If the mother decides to terminate the pregnancy, she can do so earlier with the utmost privacy and confidentiality since her pregnancy may not yet be visible.

Screening tests can give false positive results. A positive result (showing an increased risk) does not mean that your baby definitely has a health problem, but indicates that you may wish to pursue further testing options.

The first trimester detection rates for Down syndrome are 80 to 85 percent. A negative screening test is usually reassuring. It is important to understand that screening tests will not detect all cases of Down syndrome. Therefore it is still possible that a woman with a negative screen result can give birth to a child with Down syndrome.

Other chromosomal abnormalities that may be identified by Down syndrome screening:

Triploidy:

Triploidy is a common chromosomal anomaly affecting about 1% of conceptions *(Benacerraf 1999)* and over 6% of human abortions *(Eiben et al., 1990)*. Triploidy is a condition in which there are three sets of 23 chromosomes instead of the usual two so that there are 69 chromosomes in all. Most Triploidy pregnancies miscarry before 20 weeks of pregnancy and very few of the reminder reach term; the birth prevalence is less than 1 per 100 000. Of the few infants that are born, most die within a few hours or weeks *(Wald et al., 2000)*.

In Down syndrome screening programmes Triploidy pregnancies can be identified because they tend to have very high or very low levels of hCG (free β or total hCG), low levels of oestriol and high or low levels of AFP *(Canick & Saller 1993)*. Low hCG and AFP appear to be associated with Triploidy in which the prenatal origin of the extra chromosome is maternal, and high hCG and high AFP tend to be found when the origin is paternal *(Eiben et al., 1996)*. Nuchal translucency measurements also tend to be high in cases of Triploidy *(Wald et al., 2000)*.

Trisomy 18:

Trisomy 18 occurs with a birth prevalence of about one-tenth that of Down syndrome and is the second most common aneuploidy surviving to birth. In most cases survival is only for a few weeks or months since there are abnormalities affecting many organs and structures *(Wald et al., 2000)*.

In the second trimester, Serum AFP, hCG and uE3 levels are all low: AFP (0.65 MoM), uE3 (0.43 MoM), total hCG (0.36 MoM), free β-hCG (0.38 MoM) *(Hackshaw et al., 1995)*. Little has been published on inhibin levels and trisomy 18 but there is an indication that levels is about 25% lower than in unaffected pregnancies *(Hackshaw et al., 1995; Wenstrom et al., 1998; Lambert-Messerlian et al., 1998)*. In the first trimester, nuchal translucency measurement *(Sherod et al., 1997)* is increased but, given the high natural fetal loss of this condition, it is not clear how many trisomy 18 pregnancies that would progress to term have abnormal nuchal translucency measurements *(Wald et al., 2000)*.

Turner syndrome:

Turner syndrome occurs in females who lack an X chromosome in their cells, with a birth prevalence of about 1 in 2000 female newborn. As with other aneuploides there is a high fetal loss rate. Some affected individuals have structural malformations, mainly renal and cardio-vascular, but most are not seriously disabled *(Spencer et al., 2000)*.

In pregnancies with Turner syndrome associated with hydrops (cystic hygroma) serum markers show the same pattern as those in Down syndrome pregnancies (low AFP, low uE3 and high hCG levels) but in those without hydrops the hCG levels is low *(Saller et al., 1992; Canick et al., 1993)*.

It has been shown that Turner syndrome with hydrops is associated with high inhibin-A levels (3.9 MoMs) and low levels in those without hydrops (0.64 MoMs*) (Messerlian et al., 1998)*. In the first trimester, Turner syndrome is associated with increased nuchal translucency (median of 4.7 MoM) and low PAPP-A (median of 0.49 MoM), whilst free B-hCG levels were not markedly raised (median of 1.11 MoM), based on 46 cases *(Spencer et al., 2000)*.

CHAPTER 4

PRENATAL DIAGNOSIS FOR DOWN SYNDROME

Prenatal diagnosis is the process of determining the condition of a fetus before it is born. This type of diagnosis has become an important part of pregnancy care. The earliest form of prenatal testing was very simple. The mother noted fetal activity in the womb and the doctor manually felt the unborn child through the mother's abdomen. Eventually machines were developed for listening to the fetal heart beat.

Prenatal diagnosis began to improve with the development of **amniocentesis** in the 1950s. In the 1960s, the ability to culture cells from amniotic fluid was developed. Beginning in 1968, cells from amniotic fluid could be analyzed for chromosome disorders *(Gale 2006).*

Benefits of prenatal diagnosis:

The benefits of prenatal diagnosis are as follows:
1. Prenatal diagnosis determines the outcome of pregnancy.
2. It is helpful for couples to decide whether to continue the pregnancy.
3. It indicates possible complications that can arise at birth process.
4. Prenatal diagnosis is helpful for the management of remaining weeks of pregnancy.
5. It prepares the couple for the birth of a child with an abnormality.
6. Finding conditions that may affect future pregnancies.

Prenatal diagnosis can be helpful for the improvement of the outcome of pregnancy using fetal treatment *(Signh et al., 2005)*.

Prenatal diagnosis is indicated whenever there is a familial, maternal or fetal condition that confers an increased risk of a malformation, chromosome abnormality or genetic disorder. Some prenatal diagnostic studies are prompted by abnormal results of tests such as ultrasonographic examinations or maternal serum screening. In other circumstances, parents may be affected with a genetic disorder, may be carriers for autosomal recessive or X-linked recessive disorders or may be a member of an ethnic group with an increased risk of a specific genetic disease *(Cunniff 2004)*.

Indications for prenatal diagnosis had been entered into the database from the information provided on test requisition forms. In many instances, more than one indication was present. For simplicity, we reduced multiple indications to a single indication using the following priority order:
1. "fetal demise"
2. "abnormal ultrasound" (anomalies or markers)
3. "abnormal serum" screening results, including patients who were screen-positive for Down syndrome, trisomy 18, or an open neural tube defect.
4. "family history" of aneuploidy or known presence of a translocation or inversion segregating in the family.
5. "maternal age" of 35 years or older.
6. "other cases" including prenatal biochemical or molecular referrals, history of spontaneous abortion, anxiety, etc *(Benn et al., 2004)*.

112

Approximately 50% of all potentially viable Down syndrome pregnancies were diagnosed prenatally. This proportion did not seem to change substantially over the past 12 years and is less than might have been expected, given the improvements in screening over that time *(Benn et al., 2004)*.

It is important to establish whether this reflects patients attitudes toward prenatal testing, a desire not to know whether the fetus is affected or if there are substantial access barriers to the serum screening tests, advanced ultrasound services, counseling and cytogenetics *(Benn et al., 2004)*.

Ideally, prenatal aneuploidy screening would achieve levels of efficacy such that invasive testing was only needed to confirm or precisely define a chromosomal abnormality that had been established as being present by noninvasive techniques *(Benn et al., 2003)*.

Technique used in prenatal diagnosis of Down syndrome:

Non-invasive techniques:

Fetal visualization:
- Ultrasound
- Fetal echocardiography
- Magnetic resonance imaging (MRI)
- Radiography
- Screening for fetal Down syndrome:
    - Measuring MSAFP
    - Measuring maternal unconjugated estriol

113

o Measuring maternal serum beta-human chorionic gonadotropin (HCG).
- Separation of fetal cells from the mother's blood *(Signh et al., 2005).*

Invasive techniques:

Fetal visualization:
- Embryoscopy
- Fetoscopy

Fetal tissue sampling:

- Amniocentesis
- Chorionic villus sampling (CVS)
- Percutaneous umbilical blood sampling (PUBS).
- Preimplantation biopsy of blastocysts obtained by in vitro fertilization.

Cytogenetic investigations:

Detection of chromosomal aberrations:

- Fluorescent in situ hybridization
- Molecular genetic techniques *(Signh et al., 2005).*

Techniques used in prenatal diagnosis:

There are a variety of non-invasive and invasive techniques available for prenatal diagnosis of fetal abnormalities. Each of them can be applied only during specific time periods during pregnancy for greatest utility.

Table (12): Techniques used in prenatal diagnosis

Technique	Optimal time (in weeks)
Non-invasive	
Fetal cells in maternal circulation	
Preimplantation Genetic diagnosis	
Invasive	
Amniocentesis	16 weeks
Chorionic villus sampling	10-12 weeks
Percutaneous umbilical blood sample	18-22 weeks
Fetoscopy	10-12 weeks

(Muller & Young 1998)

Noninvasive prenatal diagnosis Techniques:

Separation of fetal cells from the maternal circulation:

Fetal blood cells make access to maternal circulation through the placental villi. These cells can be collected safely from approximately 18 weeks gestation onward, although by successful procedures these cells can be collected at 12 weeks gestation *(Orlandi 1990)*. The fetal cells can be sorted out and analyzed by different techniques *(Singh et al., 2005)*.

For many years the possibility of identifying fetal cells in the maternal circulation and analyzing them for the presence of trisomy 21 has offered the prospect of so-called non-invasive antenatal diagnosis *(Wald et al., 1997)*. The isolation of intact nucleated fetal cells from maternal blood and subsequent prenatal diagnoses of human aneuploides have been demonstrated previously *(Bianchi et al., 1992; Ganshirt et al., 1993; Simpson et al., 1993) (Singh et al., 2005)*.

The ratio of fetal cells to maternal cells has been shown to be higher in pregnancies associated with aneuploides but the challenge is still to identify the very few fetal cells within millions of maternal cells *(Wald et al., 2000)*.

Fluorescent in situ hybridization:

FISH uses different fluorescent-labeled probes, which are single-stranded DNA conjugated with fluorescent dyes and are specific to regions of individual chromosomes. These probes hybridize with complementary target DNA sequences

116

(Trask 1991) in the genome and can detect chromosomal abnormalities, such as trisomies *(Elias 1992),* monosomies and duplications.

Three types of DNA probes are used in FISH analysis. Whole chromosome probes are specific to a whole chromosome or a chromosome segment and are applied to metaphase spread for the identification of translocations or aneuploidy *(Singh et al., 2005).* Three fluorescent signals are seen in the presence of trisomy 21 instead of the usual two. However, this may not occur with all affected cells some times-affected cells reveal only two signals. The method is therefore less reliable than conventional diagnostic methods involving amniocentesis and the culture of fetal cells *(Wald et al., 2000).* Repetitive probes, such as alpha satellite sequences located in the centromeric regions of human chromosomes, are used in the identification of marker chromosomes and aneuploidy *(Singh et al., 2005).*

However, *Lo et al., 1998* reported that fetal DNA could be detected in maternal plasma as early as 7 weeks gestation and the concentration of fetal DNA in total maternal plasma range from 3.4% in early pregnancy to 6.2% in late pregnancy *(Wald et al., 2000).*

Zong and his colleges' (2000) reported that the amount of fetal DNA in maternal plasma is significantly elevated in pregnancies with certain fetal aneuploides (average gestational age 14 weeks).

Invasive prenatal diagnosis techniques:

Include chorionic villus sampling (CVS), amniocentesis, cordocentesis or percutaneous umbilical blood sampling (PUBS), fetal tissue sampling, as well as embryoscopy and fetoscopy.

Some diagnostic results may be obtained by more than one technique: for example, fetal karyotype can be obtained from cells from amniocentesis, chorionic villus sampling or fetal blood sampling.

First trimester screening for aneuploidy and congenital anomalies using ultrasound for fetal nuchal translucency measurements and maternal serum biochemical markers have been developed with trisomy 21 detection rate of 60 to 90% with a screen positive (false positive) of approximately 5% to 10%. Diagnostic invasive prenatal diagnosis with chorionic villus sampling at 10 to 14 weeks is offered for first trimester positive screening, while first or second trimester positive screening tests may undergo diagnostic invasive prenatal diagnosis with amniocentesis after 15 weeks *(Wilson et al., 2005)*.

Preimplantation genetic diagnosis:

Recent advances in the science of prenatal diagnosis allow for the evaluation of an affected embryo or an abnormal cell line prior to gestation within the womb via Preimplantation genetic diagnosis. The technique can use for any genetic condition, which can be detected with a chromosome-specific probe *(Jill Mauldin 2000)*.

For couples at high risk for having affected offspring, the options for prenatal diagnosis were previously limited to analyzing fetal DNA samples obtained by chorionic villus sampling or amniocentesis. However, couples then face the dilemma of whether or not to terminate the pregnancy if the genetic abnormality is present. In some cases this may not be a viable option for religious or personal reasons *(Clericuzio 2001)*.

Initially the principle indication for PGD was an inherited single gene or X-liked disorder or for the small number of couples carrying a balance translocation. Now it is carried out for the more common situation where the couple are at high a priori risk because of a having had a previous child with standard trisomy or in some services were they are simply at advanced reproductive age *(Clericuzio 2001)*.

The selection of normal embryos following PGD performed on blastomeres is not perfect and there is a residual risk of aneuploidy. An alternative PGD method based on fluorescence in-situ hybridisation (FISH) analysis of the first and second polar bodies has been developed to overcome this *(Cuckle 2005)*.

These techniques will be helpful for selective transfer and implantation of those pregnancies into the uterus that are not affected by a specific genetic disorder. This approach will be more acceptable to those couples who oppose abortions *(Singh et al., 2005)*.

In this procedure, a single cell is taken from the early embryo and analyzed by molecular techniques after DNA amplification by polymerase chain reaction. For this technique to be useful, it is essential to know the precise abnormality being sought, which usually means that both the genetic locus and the mutation have been identified in a previous child or another family member. PGD is performed in a limited number of prenatal diagnostic centers and systematic outcome analyses of large groups of patients are not available *(Cunniff 2004)*.

Chorionic villus sampling (CVS):

Chorionic villus sampling (CVS) is the most common first trimester invasive prenatal diagnosis technique for evaluation of fetal karyotype, molecular and biochemical abnormalities. CVS is an ultrasound-guided technique that is usually performed in the first trimester between 10 and 13 weeks 6 days gestation. Although the procedure was initially developed as a transcervical technique, both transcervical and transabdominal techniques are currently be used. In contrast to amniocentesis, which obtains amnioticfluid, the CVS obtains chorionic tissue from the developing placenta *(Wilson et al., 2005)*.

PROCEDURE:

Ultrasound is performed prior to CVS to determine fetal cardiac activity, gestational age, number of fetuses and uterine factors such as fibroids, amnion-chorion separation or contractions *(Wilson et al., 2005)*.

Concurrent use of ultrasound with CVS is recommended to allow continuous observation of the biopsy forceps, catheter or needle tip. Sterile technique, including sterile gloves and a procedure tray with antiseptic solution, gauze pads and sterile speculum should be used *(Wilson et al., 2005)*.

The transcervical Done at 10-12 weeks gestation chorionic villus sampling technique uses either a biopsy forceps or a flexible plastic catheter. Prior to insertion of the transcervical instrument, a speculum is placed in the vagina and the cervix and vaginal walls are cleansed with antiseptic solution. In the majority of cases, further manipulation of the uterus and cervix by a tenaculum is not necessary. Transcervical CVS utilizing the biopsy forceps requires directing the forceps through the cervix and into the placental tissue under continuous ultrasound guidance. A biopsy is performed and the forceps is gently withdrawn. Transcervical CVS utilizing the catheter requires directing the catheter, with a plastic or metal obtruder which shape can be moulded to allow the catheter to pass, attached to a 20 to 30cc syringe through the cervix and into the placental tissue under continuous ultrasound guidance. The catheter is withdrawn through the placental tissue to obtain the specimen with negative pressure by the syringe *(Wilson et al., 2005)*.

The transabdominal Done at 10 weeks gestation or later. Chorionic villus sampling technique generally utilizes a free hand technique with continuous ultrasound guidance, similar to amniocentesis or cordocentesis. Local anesthetic may be considered. A 19 or 20 gauge spinal needle is used for the transabdominal technique, while other needle options include a 2 needle set with an outer gauge of 18. The needle is moved back and forth (5-10 movements) in the placental tissue to obtain the specimen with negative pressure by the syringe. A smaller sample (pieces of villi) is taken as compared to transcervical, CVS bleeding after the procedure is rare, CVS takes approximately 5-7 minutes not including preparation time *(Wilson et al., 2005)*.

Rhesus prophylaxis is given if the woman is known to be Rhesus negative according to SOGC guidelines *(Kee et al., 2003)*. Patients are generally requested to have limited activity for 12 to 24 hours following the CVS procedure, but the efficacy of decreased activity in reducing the risk of pregnancy loss has not been well studied *(Wilson et al., 2005)*.

Advantage of CVS:

The major advantage of CVS is the earlier gestational age at sampling than amniocentesis (10-12 weeks versus 15-18 weeks) affording earlier results. If a chromosomal or DNA abnormality is detected and pregnancy termination is requested, some of the physical and emotional stresses of pregnancy termination may be less than when termination follows amniocentesis at a later gestational age.

Secondly, specific molecular diagnoses with DNA may be extracted directly from the villi, allowing an earlier result without cell culturing for these genetic disorders.

Thirdly, direct chromosomal analysis may be used in certain situations for rapid results in less than 24 hours by either cytogenetic or fluorescent in situ hybridization (FISH) techniques *(Wilson et al., 2005)*.

Disadvantages and risks of CVS:

(A) Confined Placental Mosaicism:

Confined placental mosaicism, a discrepancy between the chromosomes in the chorionic and fetal tissues, is a biologic placental factor which is present in 1% to 2% of pregnancies. Although this finding is usually limited to the placental tissue and is not usually present in the fetus, additional amniocentesis should be offered for further evaluation.

The additional procedure may increase pregnancy complication risks. Clinical effects of the confined placental mosaicism can vary depending on the specific chromosome involved. The concerns that need to be considered in this situation are uniparental disomy and risks of intrauterine growth restriction and fetal death associated with placental dysfunction *(Wilson et al., 2005)*.

(B) Maternal Contamination:

Contamination by maternal decidual tissue is possible, but this potential problem can be minimized with very careful attention to cleaning or stripping of the chorionic villi of maternal decidual cells under the dissecting microscope prior to tissue culturing. This has not been a significant problem in most cytogenetic laboratories with long-term experience in CVS *(Wilson et al., 2005)*.

(C) Pregnancy Loss:

The background risk of spontaneous pregnancy loss in the advanced maternal age group, after ultrasound has confirmed a viable pregnancy at 10 weeks gestational age when no procedure is undertaken, is estimated at 2% to 3%. The CVS procedure adds approximately 1% to 2% above the background in comparison to the 0.5 to 1% risk for amniocentesis *(Papp et al., 2002)*.

Vaginal bleeding occurring prior to the procedure increases the risk of pregnancy loss following CVS by either transcervical or transabdominal route. The risk of pregnancy loss increases with the number of attempts needed to obtain the chorionic tissue and should be limited to 2 attempts. Uterine and placental location may alter procedural risk factors depending on the CVS technique used. Uterine fibroids may cause some additional risks of technique success and pregnancy loss.

While the risks associated with transcervical technique were once thought to be double those of transabdominal technique more recent evidence demonstrates similar rates of spontaneous post-procedure pregnancy loss *(Wilson et al., 2005)*.

(D) Limb or Facial Anomalies:

The risk of limb or facial anomalies is higher if CVS is done at a gestational age earlier than nine weeks. CVS is generally restricted to greater than or equal to 10 weeks gestational age in most centres. The incidence of transverse limb defects (minor or major) in the general population is estimated at 9 in 10 000 live births. One-third of these anomalies may be due to a vascular disruption sequence event which may be associated with a CVS procedure. The risk of a limb or facial abnormality related to the CVS procedure could be as high as one in 3000 fetuses *(Froster & Jackson 1994)*. A recent report from the World Health Organization registry concluded that CVS is not associated with increased risks for fetal loss or anomalies *(Wilson et al., 2005)*.

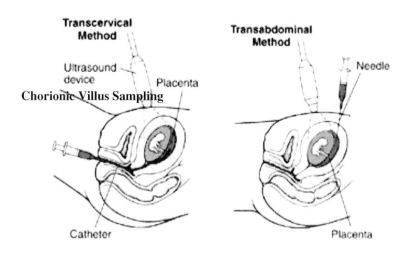

Comparison between transcervical and transabdominal chorionic villus sampling:

The transcervical technique with the biopsy forceps may be used for most placental locations, the transcervical technique with the catheter may be used for posterior placental locations, and the transabdominal technique is better suited for fundal and anterior placental locations *(Wilson et al., 2005)*.

Both the transcervical and transabdominal technique usually obtain 5 to 25 mg of chorionic tissue. This adequate amount of chorionic villus tissue is generally obtained with 1 aspiration but 2 attempts do not increase the risk of post-procedure loss.

Both transabdominal and transcervical chorionic villus sampling have similar accuracy *(Brambati et al., 1990)*; the transcervical technique is associated with a greater risk of post-procedural spotting or minimal bleeding (10%-20%) *(Shime et al., 1992)*; while the transabdominal technique has increased uterine discomfort and cramps. Infection has not been identified as a significant factor in the large number of patients having transcervical procedures *(Wilson et al., 2005)*.

Some genetic centres will use CVS techniques for both singleton and twin pregnancies. The safety and accuracy of CVS and twins is reported by a small number of centers *(Decatte et al., 1996)*; Separate instruments should be used when sampling multiple pregnancies *(Wilson et al., 2005)*.

AMNIOCENTESIS:

Amniocentesis is an ultrasound-guided invasive prenatal diagnosis procedure usually performed after 15 weeks gestational age for determination of fetal karyotype, molecular and biochemical abnormalities. The two most common tests performed on the amniotic fluid are the fetal karyotype from fetal and membrane cells in the amniotic fluid after tissue culturing or direct fluorescent insitu hybridization (FISH) techniques and direct measurement of amniotic fluid alpha fetoprotein (AFAFP). Other genetic diagnoses can be obtained by biochemical or molecular techniques after discussion with the local prenatal diagnosis centre. Results can generally be obtained prior to 20 weeks gestational age. The fetal karyotype will usually take 1 to 3 weeks from the time of amniocentesis, depending on the cytogenetic laboratory. The major disadvantage of amniocentesis is that results of the prenatal diagnosis are not available until 17 to 20 weeks gestational age. If genetic abnormalities are identified and the patient requests termination of pregnancy, the techniques of pregnancy termination such as induction of labour or dilatation and evacuation, carry a greater emotional and physical risk to the woman than a first trimester termination by dilatation and curettage *(Wilson et al., 2005)*.

PROCEDURE:

Ultrasound is performed prior to amniocentesis to determine fetal cardiac activity, fetal gestational age, location of placenta, amniotic fluid volume, number of fetuses and uterine factors such as fibroids, amnion-chorion separation or contractions. More detailed fetal anatomy may be included, depending on the centre and the age of the pregnancy *(ACOG 2001).*

The needle insertion site is identified by the ultrasound information. The skin insertion site is cleaned with an antiseptic solution. The use of local anesthetic in the abdominal wall is not generally necessary *(Alfirevic & Dadelszen 2004).*

The procedure is usually performed with a 20 to 22 gauge spinal needle using a single continuous movement of the needle through the abdominal and uterine wall. It is important that entry into the amniotic sac is a sharp thrust to avoid tenting of the amnion. A 10 to 20 cc syringe is used to aspirate the amniotic fluid following removal of the needle style. The volume of amniotic fluid removed is 15 to 30 cc and depends on the indication for prenatal diagnosis and the gestational age at the time of the procedure. The removal of the spinal needle reverses the technique used for insertion *(Wilson et al., 2005).*

Sterile technique, including sterile gloves and a procedure tray with antiseptic solution, gauze pads, forceps and sterile drape should be used. The concurrent use of ultrasound with amniocentesis is recommended to allow continuous observation of the fetus, amniotic fluid and position of the needle tip.

Although published results regarding transplacental amniocentesis have not shown significant increased risks for miscarriage *(Marthn et al., 1997),* increased risk of fetal-maternal transfusions has been reported *(Tabor et al., 1987).*

Removal of the amniotic fluid generally takes less than 1 minute. The patient may experience some mild uterine cramping and pressure sensation. The amniotic fluid is generally similar in appearance to dilate urine. Occasionally, blood-tinged amniotic fluid may be obtained, generally due to maternal bleeding into the amniotic cavity at the time of the procedure *(Alfirevic et al., 2004)*.

If the patient has previously had a history of antepartum bleeding, the amniotic fluid may be brown or dark red in colour due to blood pigments being absorbed across the chorioamnionic membranes. The presence of discolored fluid on amniocentesis is associated with an increased risk of pregnancy loss *(Alfirevic et al., 2004)*.

No more than 2 uterine needle insertions into or through the uterine wall are recommended. If the procedure is unsuccessful, further attempts can be made with a delay of at least 24 hours. Freshly blood-stained amniotic fluid should be separately analyzed by a Kleihauer test and cell count to determine whether the new blood is maternal or fetal. If the blood is fetal, the AFAFP value may be elevated without a congenital anomaly as the etiology *(Eddleman et al., 2003)*.

Rhesus prophylaxis is given if the woman is known to be Rhesus negative according to SOGC guidelines *(Kee et al., 2003)*.

Patients are generally requested to have limited activity for 12 to 24 hours following the amniocentesis procedure, but the efficacy of decreased activity in reducing the risk of pregnancy loss has not been well studied *(Wilson et al., 2005)*.

DISADVANTAGES AND RISKS OF AMNIOCENTESIS:

(A) Fetal Loss:

Fetal loss after amniocentesis is estimated to be 1 in every 100 to 600 procedures above the background loss rate *(Eddleman et al., 2003).*

(B) Infection:

The risk of infection introduced at the time of the amniocentesis is estimated to be 1 to 2 in 3000 procedures. Recent information indicates that approximately 10% to 50% of post-amniocentesis losses have evidence of low-grade infections at the time of the procedure with increased cytokine levels in the amniotic fluid *(Wilson et al., 2005).*

(C) Fetal Injury:

Serious fetal injuries at the time of amniocentesis are rare with or without continuous ultrasound guidance. Small skin dimpling lesions have been reported following contact of the fetus with the needle, but these are generally minimal and the specific anatomic location may be the only consideration *(Wilson et al., 2005).*

(D) Other Complications:

Complications without fetal loss following amniocentesis include continued leakage of amniotic fluid, bleeding and uterine irritability. These complications are estimated to occur in 1% to 5% of procedures. These complications are generally self-limited *(Sundberg et al., 1997)*. Recommendations may include bed rest, but this has not been well studied and additional serial ultrasound monitoring if continued amniotic fluid leakage is present. The benefit of antibiotic use with amniotic fluid leakage has not been evaluated. Persistent amniotic fluid leakage associated with ongoing severe oligohydramnios can lead to pulmonary hypoplasia and arthrogryposis in the newborn. Those results of the prenatal diagnosis are not available *(Wilson et al., 2005)*.

EARLY AMNIOCENTESIS:

Early amniocentesis, performed before 14 to 15 weeks gestation, potentially provides fetal chromosome results much earlier than second trimester amniocentesis. Studies have shown that the chromosome study results from early amniocentesis are as accurate as those obtained in the second trimester. In contrast to CVS, potential advantages associated with early amniocentesis include the use of a familiar technique that is widely available, the ability to assess amniotic fluid alpha-fetoprotein measurement and reduction of maternal cell contamination.

Early amniocentesis may be technically more difficult to perform because the amnion and chorion, which must be pierced by the needle, are often still separated by the extraembryonic coelom until 14 weeks gestation. This may result

130

in tenting and stretching of the amniotic membranes and prevent access to the amniotic cavity *(Clericuzio 2001)*.

Another difficulty encountered in early amniocentesis may be that the placenta is so extensive that access to the optimal pocket of fluid may require a transplacental approach. At this time, there has not been an observed increased rate of complications associated with transplacental early amniocentesis *(Clericuzio 2001)*.

Findings from the large Canadian multicentred prospective randomized trial (CEMAT 98); comparing early amniocentesis (11 to 12 weeks 6 days) and mid-trimester amniocentesis (15 to 16 weeks 6 days) have confirmed the findings from smaller randomized trials. Significant differences for early amniocentesis compared with mid-trimester amniocentesis were found for:

Total fetal losses including pre procedure, post-procedure, stillbirth and neonatal death (7.6% in the early amniocentesis group vs. 5.95% in the mid-trimester amniocentesis group, $P = 0.012$), for newborn clubfoot (1.3%, 0.1%, $P = 0.0001$) and for post-procedural amniotic fluid leakage (3.7% vs.1.5%, $P = 0.0007$). Cytogenetic culture failures were also more likely in the early amniocentesis group (1.8% for early amniocentesis vs. 0.2% for mid-trimester amniocentesis, $P < 0.0001$), requiring additional invasive prenatal diagnosis techniques for these women if further diagnosis was requested. There was no significant difference in the incidence of neonatal respiratory disease or congenital hip dislocation when comparing the 2 groups *(Philip et al., 2002)*.

131

Early amniocentesis does not appear to be appropriate for routine prenatal diagnosis at gestational ages of 11 to 13 weeks 6 days gestation. A recent randomized trial evaluated the safety and accuracy of amniocentesis and transabdominal chorionic villus sampling (CVS) performed at 11 to 14 weeks of gestation *(Philip et al., 2002)*.

There were 3775 women randomized into 2 groups (1914 to CVS; 1861 to amniocentesis). The primary outcome measure of a composite of fetal loss plus preterm delivery before 28 weeks of gestation in cytogenetically normal fetuses was similar for both groups (2.1% for CVS vs. 2.3% for amniocentesis, P = NS). Spontaneous pregnancy losses before 20 weeks and procedure-related indicated termination appeared increased in the amniocentesis groups (RR 1.74, 95% CI, 0.94-3.22, P =.07). There was a 4.65-fold increase in the rate of talipes equinovarus after early amniocentesis (95% CI, 1.01-21.5, P = 0.017). The study concluded that amniocentesis at 13 weeks carries a significantly increased risk of talipes equinovarus compared with CVS and a possible increase in early unintended pregnancy loss *(Wilson et al., 2005)*.

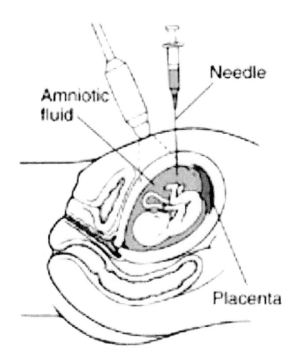

Amniotic fluid

Needle

Placenta

Amniocentesis

Percutaneous Umbilical Blood Sampling (PUBS):

PUBS is also known as cordocentesis *(Daffos 1985)*. It is a method for fetal blood sampling and is performed after 16 weeks gestation. It is the most accurate method used to confirm the results of CVS or amniocentesis. It is routinely used in the management of Rhesus isoimmunization and can be used to obtain samples for chromosome analysis. The tissue is tested for the presence of extra material from chromosome 21 for diagnosis of Down syndrome. PUBS can not be done until the 18-22 and week. It carries the greatest risk of miscarriage *(Singh et al., 2005)*.

A needle is inserted into the umbilical cord under ultrasound guidance and fetal blood is collected from the umbilical vein for chromosome analysis. This technique is also useful for evaluating fetal metabolism and hematologic abnormalities *(Singh et al., 2005)*.

While fetal blood sampling has been obtained, the umbilical vein is preferred because it is larger and is less likely to cause fetal bradycardia when punctured. In order to confirm that the sample is fetal in origin, the mean corpuscular volume (MCV) of the sample should be assessed. The MCV of a sample of fetal blood should be above 100 fL *(Clericuzio 2001)*.

Complications / risks of percutaneous umbilical blood sampling:

The most critical factor related to the safety of the procedure is operator experience. Reported fetal loss rates for PUBS are 7.2% (96/1328) overall and 3% in a low risk group (20/660). In addition to fetal loss, other complications associated with PUBS include bleeding from the puncture site in the umbilical cord, cord hematomas, transient fetal bradycardia, infection and feto-maternal hemorrhage *(Clericuzio 2001).*

Bleeding from the cord puncture site is the most common complication and is usually self-limited. Fetal bradycardia, which lasted for a short time in the majority of cases, occurred after 9% of the procedures. In a report on diagnostic cordocentesis and intravascular transfusions, bleeding was observed from the umbilical cord puncture site in 29% of cases. Although the duration of bleeding was significantly longer after arterial puncture than after puncture of the umbilical vein, the blood loss was not clinically significant in any of the cases. The incidence of a clinically significant fetal bradycardia was 6.6% *(Clericuzio 2001).*

Clinical uses of PUBS:

Based on the available data, it is clear that PUBS is a riskier procedure than CVS or amniocentesis. Currently, PUBS is offered only where there is no alternative to achieve a timely diagnosis. Fortunately, there have been major inroads in cytogenetic, molecular and ultrasound techniques that have diminished the need for fetal blood based diagnosis. For example, the use of PUBS for rapid fetal chromosome analysis for trisomies 13, 18, and 21 has been largely replaced by fluorescence in situ hybridization (FISH) techniques applied to amniocytes, which can provide chromosome results within 48 hours. Placental biopsy carries a very low risk and villi obtained throughout gestation can be processed within 48 hours *(Clericuzio 2001).*

135

Fetal visualization:

Embryoscopy:

Embryoscopy is performed in the first trimester of pregnancy *(Cullen 1990)*. In this technique, a rigid endoscope is inserted via the cervix in the space between the amnion and the chorion, under sterile conditions and ultrasound guidance, to visualize the embryo for the diagnosis of structural malformations *(Singh et al., 2005)*.

Fetoscopy:

Fetoscopy is performed during the second trimester. In this technique, a fine-caliber endoscope is inserted into the amniotic cavity through a small maternal abdominal incision, under sterile conditions and ultrasound guidance, for the visualization of the embryo to detect the presence of subtle structural abnormalities. It also is used for fetal blood and tissue sampling. Fetoscopy is associated with a 3-5% risk of miscarriage; therefore, it is superseded by detailed ultrasound scanning *(Singh et al., 2005)*.

CHAPTER 5

FACTORS AFFECTING DOWN SYNDROME RISK EVALUATION

Several factors interfere with levels of maternal serum alpha fetoprotein (AFP), human chorionic gonadotrophin (hCG) and unconjugated estriol (uE3), the three markers used for Down syndrome (DS); and this can influence the final risk evaluation and thus Down syndrome screening performance. These factors include maternal weight *(Wald et al., 1981)*, ethnic group *(Macri et al., 1976)*, multiparity *(Mooney et al., 1994)*, presence of insulin-dependent diabetes *(Reece et al., 1987)* and previous affected pregnancies *(Stene et al., 1984)*. Other factors include smoking *(Cuckle et al., 1990)* and probably alcohol or drug consumption *(Barclay & Lie 2007)*.

Gestational age:

Maternal age older than 35 years at the time of delivery has historically been used to identify women at risk of having a child with Down syndrome, and these women have been offered genetic counseling and amniocentesis or chorionic villus sampling *(Barclay & Lie 2007)*.

However, tests are now available to screen younger women using maternal serum alpha-fetoprotein levels, hCG and unconjugated estriol (triple screen) to improve the detection rate of Down syndrome to 70%. Levels of the triple markers are reduced when the fetus has trisomy 18 and adding inhibin A to quadruple screen improves the Down syndrome detection rate to 80% *(Barclay & Lie 2007)*.

137

Nuchal translucency measurement can also be used to detect fetal chromosomal, genetic, structural abnormalities and systematic measurement guidelines have now been standardized and can be combined with two first-trimester serum markers (free β-hCG, and PAPPA-A). The uses of screening for chromosomal abnormalities have reduced the number of amniocenteses performed and, therefore, the resulting fetal losses *(Barclay & Lie 2007)*.

Maternal weight:

For each of the analytes, levels are on average higher in lighter weight women and lower in heavier weight women. Adjusting maternal weight provides only minimal improvement in Down syndrome screening. However, weight adjustments should be performed for other reasons. AFP levels should be adjusted when screening for open neural tube defects and AFP, μE3 and hCG levels should be adjusted when screening for trisomy 18. Laboratories should utilize published weight adjustment formulas only until in-house data are collected and new laboratory-specific formulas derived *(Palomaki et al., 2006)*.

Serum AFP, uE3 and hCG concentrations change with maternal weight. A summary of the literature **(Table 12)** show that, on average, for a 20 kg increase in weight serum AFP decreases by about 17%, uE3 decreases by about 7%, and hCG decreases by about 16% *(Haddow et al., 2004)*.

Table (13): Median serum marker levels according to maternal weight

| Median MoM for | | | Number of | Maternal |
hCG	uE3	AFP	women	weight
1.13	1.09	1.09	172	<50
1.16	1.04	1.12	215	50-54
1.11	0.99	1.04	366	55-59
1.04	0.99	0.99	346	60-64
0.92	0.95	0.93	290	65-69
0.91	0.99	0.84	165	70-74
1.00	0.89	0.83	129	75-79
0.82	0.87	0.80	206	$\geq$80

(Haddow et al., 2004)

Insulin-dependent diabetes:

Gestational diabetes is far more common than insulin dependent diabetes. Current information suggests that maternal serum AFP concentrations are altered only when a woman with diabetes is insulin dependent prior to pregnancy and adjustments should be only made in this situation. Maternal serum AFP levels in women who develop diabetes during pregnancy (gestational diabetes) appear not to be different than the non-diabetic population, even if insulin is subsequently required *(Sanakan & Bartels 2001).*

Several studies have studied the maternal serum concentrations of unconjugated estriol (uE3) and human chorionic gonadotropin (hCG) in women with insulin dependent diabetes (IDD). On average, MoM levels of uE3 and hCG, and are 8% and 7% lower, respectively, in women with IDD. These differences are small, and adjustments will have little impact on the resulting Down syndrome risk. This is because lower uE3 levels *increase* risk while lower hCG values *decrease* risk *(Morris et al., 2002)*.

In a series of 55 IDD pregnancies screened at the Foundation for Blood Research, 7.7% had second trimester risks of 1:270 or greater when only AFP was adjusted for IDD. After adjusting uE3 and hCG for IDD, the rate remained at 7.7%. This rate is higher than our general screen positive rate because women with IDD are somewhat older *(Morris et al., 2002)*.

Reports of the effect of insulin dependent diabetes mellitus (IDDM) on Dimicron Inhibin-A (DIA) results are more variable, ranging from 0.91 MoM to 1.17 MoM (weighted average of 1.06 MoM). Given this lack of consensus, it would be reasonable to defer adjusting DIA values for diabetic status *(Sanakan & Bartels 2001)*.

Two population-based studies have examined the birth prevalence of Down syndrome in women with IDD. Unfortunately, neither study took maternal age into account. The first surveyed 47 published data sets from 1945 through 1965 and found 7 cases of Down syndrome among 7,101 IDD pregnancies (1:1,420). This was significantly lower than the 1:955 found in 431,764 controls. This might be due to a high proportion of early onset diabetics who may have been encouraged to have their pregnancies at an earlier age *(Morris et al., 2002)*.

140

The second study found 2 cases of Down syndrome in 733 IDD pregnancies, an incidence of 1:367. However, the numbers were too small to draw any reliable conclusions *(Holding 2002)*.

A third study of 139 Down syndrome pregnancies found a two-fold increased rate of IDD among the mothers delivering babies with Down syndrome *(Palomaki et al., 1994)*. *Because* of the small numbers of affected pregnancies and the fact that most studies did not account for maternal age, there is no compelling evidence that the birth rate of Down syndrome to women with IDD is substantially different from that in non-diabetic women *(Sanakan & Bartels 2001)*.

After weight correction, AFP is about 10% lower in these women, uE3 is 7% lower, free α-hCG is 11% lower, and inhibin A is 9% lower *(Wald et al., 1996)*. The etiology of the lower levels in this disorder is not known, but may be related to vascular changes in the placenta *(Holding 2002)*.

The differences are statistically significant and can therefore usefully be taken into account in screening. There were no significant differences for total hCG and free β-hCG.

Table (14): Median serum marker levels in pregnant women with and without insulin-dependent diabetes mellitus

Serum marker	Number of women		Median MoM in diabetic women	
	Non-diabetic	Diabetic	Non weight corrected	weight corrected
AFP	252	126	0.77	0.82
uE3	252	126	0.92	0.94
Total hCG	252	126	0.95	1.00
Free α-hCG	252	126	0.86	0.89
Free β-hCG	251	126	0.96	1.01
Inhibin A	251	126	0.88	0.91

(Morris et al., 2002)

Influence of maternal smoking on Down syndrome risk evaluation:

Maternal cigarette smoking is associated with alterations in maternal serum analytes used in screening for trisomy 21 during the second trimester of pregnancy *(Spencer 1998; Ferriman et al., 1999)*. Expectant mothers who smoke have higher levels of maternal serum AFP and lower levels of uE3 and hCG than non-smoking mothers. Cuckle et al. 1990 first identified a strong link between smoking and low levels of hCG as shown in **table (14)** *(Saltvedt et al., 2006)*.

This was confirmed by Palomaki et al. *(Palomaki et al., 1993)* who showed a significant dose-response relationship between nicotine levels and decrease in hCG Multiples of Medians (MoM) in a population whose Down syndrome prevalence was significantly different between smokers and non-smokers *(Saltvedt et al., 2006)*.

The biochemical markers changes described are also consistent with findings of changes in placental morphology in the early first trimester *(Jauniaux & Burton 1992)* in which synctiotrophoblastic necrosis is increased in the placenta of smokers which may result in decreased synthesis of placental proteins (such as PAPP-A and free β-hCG) and increased permeability to fetal products such as alpha-feto protein (AFP). Such findings may be an explanation for the change in maternal serum marker levels in women who smoke *(Jaques et al., 2007)*.

Table (15): The median serum marker levels in smoking and non smoking pregnant women

Serum marker	Median MoM	
	Non-smoker	**Smoker**
AFP	0.99	1.06
uE3	1.00	0.95
Total hCG	1.02	0.91

(Malone & D'alton 2003)

Ethnic group:

The serum markers differ in concentration according to ethnic group, and these differences vary depending on whether the levels are adjusted for maternal weight *(Watt et al., 1996)*. In the screening program at St. Bartholomews Hospital, Afro-Caribbean women were, on average, heavers than Caucasian women and Asian women were, on average, lighter than Caucasian women *(Jaques et al., 2007)*.

Weight-adjusted AFP values were, on average, 22% higher in Afro-Caribbean women than in Caucasian women, Total hCG and free β-hCG were 19% and 12% higher, respectively, uE3, MoMs were approximately the same as inhibin-A and free α-hCG were both 8% lower *(Malone & d'alton 2003)*.

144

In Asian women, AFP and free β-hCG levels, on average, 6% and 9% lower than Caucasian women, uE3 and total hCG were 7% and 6% higher, respectively, inhibin A and free α-hCG levels were similar. Despite these differences, adjustment for ethnic group has a small effect on screening performance but will give a more precise estimate of risk for each individual woman screened; about 0.5% extra at a 5% false-positive rate in a population consisting equally of black and white or South Asian and white women *(Jaques et al., 2007)*.

Vaginal bleeding:

Despite its being associated with higher serum AFP levels, adjusting for vaginal bleeding is of little proven benefit *(Cuckle & van Oudgaarden et al., 1994)* and is complex, as locally derived parameters are essential *(Holding 1997)*. Furthermore, the situation is complicated by the fact that in pregnancies unaffected by Down syndrome vaginal bleeding and high AFP are independent risk factors for fetal loss, *(Haddow et al., 1986)* and the incidence of bleeding increases with maternal age *(Holding 2002)*.

Number of previous pregnancies:

Advanced maternal age is strongly associated with an increased risk of Down syndrome; however, other risk factors are less well established. Investigators from several studies have reported a positive association between parity and Down syndrome *(Kallen 1997)*, although several other groups did not find an association *(Haddow & Palomaki 1994)*. The interpretation of many of these studies has been hindered by certain methodological issues *(Lilford 1997)*. Because parity is closely correlated with maternal age, and because several early studies examining the relation between parity and Down syndrome used broad (5-year) categories in

145

controlling for maternal age *(Eidelman et al., 1988),* it has been suggested that at least part of the apparent effect of parity is due to residual confounding *(Lilford 1997).*

Additionally, there is some evidence that women of higher parity are less likely to undergo prenatal screening for Down syndrome by amniocentesis or chorionic villus sampling *(Kallen 1997)* and therefore are less likely to choose to terminate a Down syndrome pregnancy than women of lower parity. This would result in an excess of Down syndrome live births among multiparous women, even in the absence of a true biologic association with parity *(Rose et al., 2003).*

Total hCG is negatively associated with parity, decreasing by about 3% for each previous birth. The reason for this decline is not known. The effect on screening performance of adjusting hCG levels is negligible. At false-positive rate of 5%, the detection rate would increase by only 0.1%. It is, therefore, not worth while adjusting MoM values for the number of previous pregnancies. **Table (15)** shows the effect of the number of previous pregnancies on serum marker levels. All studies are corrected for maternal weight *(Rose et al., 2003).*

Table (16): Effect of the number of previous pregnancies on serum markers levels in the second trimester of pregnancy

Serum marker	Median MoM according to number of previous pregnancies				
	0	1	2	3	≥4
AFP	1.01	0.99	1.02	0.98	1.04
uE3	1.01	0.98	0.99	1.00	1.04
Total hCG	1.04	1.01	0.96	0.94	0.92
Free α-hCG	1.00	0.97	1.07	0.99	0.99
Free β-hCG	1.00	0.97	1.03	1.00	1.04
Inhibin A	1.02	0.97	1.04	1.04	1.09

(Rose et al., 2003)

Twin pregnancies:

The current concept is that first trimester NT measurement is superior to second trimester serum screening for multiple pregnancies *(Maymon et al., 2005).*

All monochromic pregnancies are monozygotic. On the other hand, most but not all dichorionic pregnancies are dizygotic. For a dizygous twin pregnancy, the risk of Down syndrome for each fetus is independent of the risk of the other. This implies that for dichorionic twin pregnancies, the pregnancy specific risk calculated by summing the individual risk estimates for each *(Meyers et al., 1997).*

On the other hand, in monochorionic pregnancies, the risk is based on an average of likelihood ratios derived from NT measurements of both twins. Therefore, diagnosis of chorionicity should be the first step in ultrasound evaluation of twins during the first trimester, and it has major implications on the noninvasive screening for aneuploidy in twins *(Weisz & Rodeck 2006).*

First trimester scanning and measurement of NT enable the identification of a fetus- specific risk for Down syndrome in dichorionic pregnancies. In twin pregnancies, the sensitivity of fetal nuchal translucency thickness in screening for trisomy 21 is similar to that in singleton pregnancies, but the specificity in monochorionic pregnancies is lower because translucency is also increased in chromosomally normal monochorionic twin pregnancies *(Sebire et al., 1996).*

In another small study, a detection rate (DR) of 100% was achieved with screen positive results of 4.3% *(Maymon et al., 2001)*. The use of first trimester combined test *(Spencer & Nicolaides 2003)* can lower the false positive rate (FPR) of NT measurement. It is estimated that by using 'pseudo- risk' and not specific risk figures, the integrated test can reach a DR5 of 78 and 93% for dichorionic and monochorionic twin pregnancies, respectively *(Wald et al., 2003)*.

Three major national studies (SURUSS, BUN and FASTER Trial) as well as many local studies *evaluated by Nicolaides 2004* demonstrate that the first trimester combined test is equivalent or superior to second trimester serum screening *(Simpson 2005)*.

A "pseudo risk" is calculated by dividing the observed MoM value in twin pregnancies by the median MoM value in twin pregnancies without Down syndrome. This is not true risk but it will have the effect of keeping the false-positive rate in twin pregnancies the same as that in singleton pregnancies. Women may be classified as screen positive or screen negative using the same cut-off level used for singleton pregnancies but without reporting a risk estimate *(Palomaki et al., 2005)*.

Serum marker levels in women with twin pregnancies might be expected to be about twice those in singleton pregnancies. This, infact observed, although some markers have levels a little greater (for example, AFP) and some a little less (for example, uE3) *(Maymon et al., 2005)*.

Assisted reproduction (ovulation induction and in vitro fertilization):

There is a suggestion that serum marker levels are affected by assisted reproduction using either ovulation induction or *in vitro* fertilization *(Muller et al., 1993; Barkai et al., 1996; Ribbet et al., 1996)*. In women who had "ovulation induction" hCG levels were, on average, 9% higher and uE3 levels were 8% lower. There was no difference for AFP *(Weisz & Rodeck 2006)*.

In women who had "in vitro fertilization" a weighted geometric mean of marker levels showed that there was no significant effect on AFP levels (median MoM 0.96%). There was suggestion that uE3 levels were low (median MoM 0.92). The effect on marker levels is insufficient to warrant adjustment in risk estimation *(Weisz & Rodeck 2006)*.

Pregnancies conceived by ART carry a higher psychological and financial burden compared to spontaneous pregnancies *(Oddens et al., 1999)*. The uptake of amniocentesis in ART pregnancies is believed to be lower compared to controls, mainly due to the inherent risks of amniocentesis in these 'more precious' pregnancies *(Geipel et al., 2004)*. Therefore, those population gains specifically from the low OAPR of the integrated test, which reduces their risk of being high risk for trisomy 21 and having an invasive test. Other issues, which apply to ART pregnancies, are:

i. A relatively older population of pregnant women,

ii. Differences in serum markers compared to spontaneous pregnancies and

iii. A higher rate of multi- fetal pregnancies *(Weisz & Rodeck 2006)*.

150

Initial studies reported a significant difference in the level of second trimester biochemical markers between IVF patients and spontaneous pregnancies *(Wald et al., 1999).* Evaluating 152 IVF pregnancies in which AFP, uE3, free hCG and total hCG were measured, median uE3 levels were 6% lower, median free hCG 9% higher and median total hCG 14% higher (all statically significant) in IVF pregnancies compared with controls. These results might explain the higher FPR in IVF pregnancies, which is about twice as high as that in controls *(Barkai et al., 1996).*

High hCG levels may be explained partly by a grater number of corpora lutea *(Frishman et al., 1997)*, by multiple implantation sites or by progesterone supplementation, which increases placental hCG *production (Weisz & Rodeck 2006).*

Alternatively, it may represent placentation failure that could result in changes in trophoblast function and thus hCG production *(Raty et al., 2003).* The low uE3 levels remain unexplained. It was suggested that in Down syndrome screening in IVF pregnancies, hCG and uE3 values should adjusted to avoid the high screen positive rate. A recent multi-center study analysis 1515 singleton pregnancies by assisted reproduction techniques (ART) found a similar trend of 12% lower uE3, 7% higher hCG and 6% lower AFP, but these differences were not significant. In this study, the FPR did not differ from age-matched controls *(Muller et al., 2003).* This might suggest that the significance found by *Wald et al., 1999* was a type I error. Other comparative studies show that serum levels of all three second trimester markers in ART pregnancies do not differ from controls *(Rice et al., 2005).*

The effect of ART on the first trimester screening is also controversial. Some studies show an increase in hCG levels *(Niemimaa et al., 2001)* and a decrease in PAPP-A or FPR between ART and spontaneous pregnancies *(Wojdemann et al., 2001)*. Interestingly, some recent studies found increased NT in ART pregnancies (MoM, multiples of median) *(Maymon & Shylman 2004; Hui et al., 2005)*.

The effect of ART on integrated (first and second trimester) screening was assessed in a group that underwent a serial disclosure Down syndrome screening program *(Maymon & Shylman 2004)*. The rate of first trimester screening FPR was comparable to controls. The rate of second trimester FPR was two- fold higher in ART group. It was concluded that ART singleton patients should be screened either by the combined or by the integrated tests *(Maymon & Shylman 2004)*. To conclude, it is postulated that Down syndrome screening in ART pregnancies is associated with a higher FPR. To decrease the magnitude of such uncertain experience, it is advised to use better screening modalities, such as the combined or integrated tests *(Weisz & Rodeck 2006)*.

CHAPTER 6

COUNSELING OF DOWN SYNDROME

Genetic counseling is a process of communication between patients and trained professionals intended to provide patients who have a genetic disease - or risk of such a disease - with information about their condition and its effect on their family. This allows patients and their families to make informed reproductive and other medical decisions *(Braithwaite et al., 2006).*

Genetic counseling can help parents balance the risks, limitations, and benefits of prenatal screening and diagnostic testing. The counseler will evaluate medical problems or risks present in a family, analyze and explain inheritance patterns of any disorders found, provide information about management and treatment of these disorders, and discuss available options with the family or individual. Two tests are available to definitively diagnose Down syndrome: chorionic villus sampling and amniocentesis *(Laurino et al., 2005).*

According to the American College of Medical Genetics, an important issue in genetic testing is defining the scope of informed consent. The obligation to counsel and obtain consent is inherent in the clinician-patient and investigator-subject relationships. In the case of most genetic tests, the patient or subject should be informed that the test might yield information regarding a carrier or disease state that requires difficult choices regarding their current or future health, insurance coverage, career, marriage, or reproductive options *(Hampel et al., 2004).*

153

The objective of informed consent is to preserve the individual's right to decide whether to have a genetic test. This right includes the right of refusal, should the individual decide the potential harm outweighs the potential benefits *(Schwind et al., 2005).*

Aims of counseling:

Genetic counseling is a health care service aimed at helping individuals and families understand the science of genetics and how it may relate to them. Genetic counselors are health care professionals certified by the American Board of Genetic Counseling aims to appreciate the values of the patient and incorporate those values into the counseling and facilitated decision making components that are vital to effective services *(Graves & Miller 2007).*

The counselor's role is to provide an unbiased, complete and accurate view of the situation, the nature of the birth defect being investigated, and what — in practical terms — its occurrence would mean for all involved *(Shafi et al., 2007).*

Counseling Aspects:

i. *Information:* In order to make an informed decision, women should be offered a clear and simple verbal explanation, supported by appropriate literature, describing options available, risks of Down syndrome and risks of screening and diagnostic procedures, including false negative rates *(Hampel et al., 2004).*

ii. ***Counseling:*** All women at risk should have timely access to sympathetic and accurate non-directive counseling before and after prenatal diagnosis and if necessary before and after termination of pregnancy *(Hampel et al., 2004).*

iii. ***Record keeping:*** Details of offers of prenatal screening and diagnosis, confirmation of diagnosis and outcome of pregnancy should be recorded in the antenatal notes *(Bennett et al., 2002).*

iv. ***Confirmation:*** Accuracy of prenatal diagnosis by cytogenetic diagnosis of terminated fetus should be confirmed *(Bennett et al., 2002).*

Assessment of the risk of Down syndrome begins with the first prenatal visit. All forms of prenatal testing for Down syndrome must be voluntary. A nondirective approach should be used when discussing the methods of prenatal screening and diagnostic testing *(Abramsky 1994).* Informed consent to testing should be documented in the patient's chart *(Newberger 2000).*

Consultation with a medical geneticist or a genetic counseler should be sought if there has been a previous pregnancy complicated by a chromosome abnormality or if either parent is known to carry a balanced translocation. Women who will be 35 years or older are on their due date should be offered chorionic villus sampling or second-trimester amniocentesis. These patients may be offered maternal serum screening and ultrasound evaluation before they make a decision about having amniocentesis, provided that they are informed of the limited sensitivity of noninvasive testing *(ACOG 1996).*

155

Women younger than 35 years should be offered maternal serum screening at 15 to 18 weeks' gestation. They should be counseled about the imperfect sensitivity of maternal serum screening and the possibility that a false-positive result could lead to invasive testing. Test results should be reported to the patient promptly. Patients who receive news of abnormal results often experience considerable anxiety *(Green 1994)*. These patients can be reassured by the knowledge that the likelihood of Down syndrome is small, even after a positive triple test *(Reynolds et al., 1993)*. Ultrasound and amniocentesis should be offered. The risk of fetal loss from amniocentesis should be discussed *(Newberger 2000)*.

If diagnostic testing reveals fetal trisomy 21, the parents should be provided with current, accurate information about Down syndrome and assistance in deciding on a course of action. Their options include continuing the pregnancy and raising the child, continuing the pregnancy and seeking adoption placement for the child or terminating the pregnancy *(Stein et al., 1997)*.

Consultation with a genetic counseler, a medical geneticist or a developmental pediatrician can be helpful to address the parents' concerns and facilitate their decision-making process *(Stein et al., 1997)*.

Parents who decide to continue the pregnancy should be advised that there is an increased risk of fetal demise in trisomy 21 pregnancies. A fetal echocardiogram should be performed at 20 weeks of gestation to detect serious cardiac malformations. An ultrasound examination should be performed at 28 to 32 weeks of gestation to monitor growth and detect duodenal atresia *(Stein et al., 1997)*. The parents should be provided with referrals to support groups and organizations that advocate for persons with Down syndrome and their families *(Saenz 1999)*.

A positive outlook should be encouraged, recognizing that improvements in medical care, early intervention, special education and vocational counseling have enabled persons with Down syndrome to live more normal lives *(Stein et al., 1997)*.

Pre-test counseling:

The family physician's best chance of avoiding these adverse consequences is by discussing the nature, purpose, and risks of screening with the patient. This discussion should include possible psychological effects of the screening test and amniocentesis, the positive and negative attributes of Down syndrome, and the patient's feelings about abortion. The family physician might be better able to provide this counseling than a genetic counselor because of experience with and knowledge of the family, but the physician must be careful not to be directive. The goal of genetic counseling is nondirective education for which genetic counselors have specific training *(Palomaki et al., 2005)*.

In a survey of physicians on how they would counsel a couple about prenatal diagnosis of a genetic disorder, one half of the physicians felt comfortable counseling and one half did not and would refer. Family physicians were more likely than obstetricians to discuss a prenatal diagnosis with a patient rather than refer her to a specialist. On the other hand, when compared with other specialists, family physicians and internists were more likely to give their opinions about abortion *(Haddow et al., 2004)*.

157

Physicians or genetic counselors might express their opinion directly or in a covert manner by focusing attention on prenatal risks and the consequences of genetic disease. For example, directive counseling can occur when the physician focuses on the negative or positive side of Down syndrome, influencing a patient's choice of abortion *(Knight & Palomaki 2003)*. It is important in nondirective counseling that the physician recognizes how his or her feelings about abortion or Down syndrome might influence a patient's decision making *(Morris et al., 2002)*. If a bias does exist, referral to a genetic counselor for pretest counseling is warranted *(Palomaki et al., 2005)*.

Regional genetics networks might also have written patient and physician information on the multiple marker screening test. The screening information should include material geared to the reading level of the physician's patient population. Anxiety regarding the test has been shown to decrease and knowledge improves when patients are given written information about the multiple marker screening tests *(Palomaki et al., 2005)*.

During the visit the physician should ascertain the patient's resources, values, expectations, and knowledge level. The counselor's job is to facilitate the process of patient decision making. The physician should elicit any questions about the test and be attentive to the emotional state of the patient. The physician can begin by describing that the goal of screening is to detect Down syndrome before birth and can then review with the patient what she knows about Down syndrome and clarify any misconceptions *(Malone & D'alton 2003)*.

The patient needs to know the screening test is not a diagnostic test but a blood test that can predict her chances of carrying a Down syndrome infant. Only amniocentesis can determine whether her baby does or does not have this disorder. The multiple marker test is excellent at ruling out Down syndrome (eg, if the test result is negative, it is likely to be a true negative). Its average detection rate is 56%, and the false-positive rate is 7% (*Palomaki et al., 2005*).

The physician should ask the patient whether she would obtain an amniocentesis to confirm a positive test. She needs to be informed that there is a chance (1% or less) of miscarriage related to the amniocentesis. Those who strongly state that under no circumstances would they undergo amniocentesis might prefer to decline testing (*Haddow et al., 2004*).

If the patient desires testing but is not sure about amniocentesis, she might experience increased anxiety during the remainder of the pregnancy if she has a positive test result but decides not to have amniocentesis. After counseling a pregnant woman, a questionnaire to assess knowledge about maternal screening will help determine what information might not have been understood. A patient can be offered   a follow-up appointment to discuss test results and to help alleviate any anxiety she might feel, particularly after a positive test (*Haddow et al., 2004*).

Post-test counseling:

The first step after a positive test result is to review the information (maternal weight, age, race, the presence of insulin-dependent diabetes mellitus, and gestational age) submitted to the laboratory with the blood sample. If this information is accurate, the next step is to order   a sonogram to verify dates of conception and confinement. If a sonogram has been done, and the estimated date of confinement is within 2 weeks of the date based on the last menstrual period, the sonogram should not be repeated *(Palomaki et al., 2005).*

In posttest counseling, a positive test result can be put into perspective for the patient immediately. For example, a 30-year-old woman with a positive test result has a 1% (or 1 in 100) chance that it was a true positive, whereas a 44-year-old woman with a positive test result has a 3.8% (or 1 in 26) chance that it was a true positive. Most laboratories provide a patient risk estimate rather than just reporting whether the test result is positive or negative. This more accurate risk estimate should be used in counseling the patient. All patients receiving a positive test result should be referred to a genetic *(Palomaki et al., 2005).*

References:

- **Abramsky L (1994):** Counseling prior to prenatal testing. In: Abramsky L, Chapple J, eds. prenatal diagnosis: the human side. *New York: Chapman & Hall, 1994:70-85.*

- **ACOG (1996):** American College of Obstetricians and Gynecologists. Maternal serum screening. *ACOG Educational Bulletin, 1996; no. 228.*

- **ACOG (2001):** Prenatal diagnosis of fetal chromosomal abnormalities. *Obstet Gynecol. 97(5 pt 1): suppl 1-2, May 2001.*

- **ACOG (2004):** first- trimester screening for fetal aneuploidy. **ACOG committee opinion No. 296:** *Obestet Gynecol 2004; 104: 215- 7.*

- **ACOG (2007): ACOG Practice Bulletin No. 77:** Screening for fetal chromosomal abnormalities. *Obstet Gynecol 2007; 109:217-28.* Gynecological Association.

- **ACOG (2008):** ACOG'S screening guide lines on chromosomal abnormalities. What they mean to patients and physicians San Diego.

- **Adams MM, Erickson JD, Layde PM & Okley GP (1981):** Down syndrome. Recent trends in the United States. *JAMA 246: 758-760.*

- **Agarwal R (2003):** Prenatal diagnosis of chromosomal anomalies: Pictorial essay. *Indian J Radiol Imaging 2003: 173-188.*

- **Alfirevic Z & Von Dadelszen P (2004):** Instruments for chorionic villus sampling for prenatal diagnosis (Cochrane Review). In the Cochrane Library, Issue 3, 2004 Chichester, UK: *John Wiley & Sons, Ltd.*

- **Alfirevic Z, Sundberg K & Brigham S (2004):** Amniocentesis and chorionic villus sampling for prenatal diagnosis (Cochrane Review). In the Cochrane Library, Issue 3, 2004. Chichester, UK: *John Wiley & Sons, Ltd.*

- **Amudha S, Aruna N & Rajangam S (2005):** Consanguinity and chromosomal abnormality. *Indian Journal of Human Genetics May-Augest 2005. vol.11, issue 2.*

- **Anderson (2005):** First- trimester screening for Down syndrome. The American college of cardiology and cardio source.*med scape cardiology Appl Radiol 2005; 34(9): 8- 18.*

161

- **Anonymous (2000):** AFP or PAPP – A. Down screening *News 2000, p41.*

- **Avgidou K, Papageorghiou A, Bindra R, Spencer K & Nicolaides KH (2005):** Prospective first-trimester screening for trisomy 21 in 30,564 pregnancies. *Am J Obstet Gynecol 2005; 192: 1761- 7.*

- **Barclay L & Lie D (2007):** New Guidelines Recommend Universal Prenatal Screening for Down syndrome. *Obstet Gynecol. 2007; 109:217-228.*

- **Barclay L & Lie D (2008):** New guidelines Recommend Universal Prenatal screening For Down syndrome CME/CE. *Medscape medical news 2007.*

- **Barkai G, Arbuzova S, Berkenstadt M, Heifetz S & Cuckle H (2003):** Frequency of Down syndrome and neural-tube defects in the same family. *Lancet 2003; 361:1331-1335.*

- **Barnhart K & Osheroff J (1998):** Follicle stimulating hormone as a predictor of fertility. *Cur. Opinion Obs. Gyn., 10, 227–232.*

- **Beaman JM & Goldie DJ (2001):** Second trimester screening for Down syndrome: 7 years experience. *J Med Screen 2001; 8:128-131.*

- **Benacerraf BR, Harlow BL & Frigoletto FD (1990):** Hypoplasia of the middle phalanx of the fifth digit: a feature of the second trimester fetuses with Down syndrome. *J Ultrasound Med 9: 389-94.*

- **Benacerraf BR (1996):** The second- trimester fetus with Down syndrome: detection using sonographic features. *Ultrasound Obstet. Gynecol. 7: 147-155.*

- **Benacereaf BR (1999):** Second trimester sonographic features of aneuploidy. In Rodeck CH & Whittle MS *(eds) Fetal Medicine. Basic Science and Clinical Practice.* London: *Churchill Livingstone, pp 553-572.*

- **Benacerraf BR (2000):** Should sonographic screening for fetal Down syndrome is applied to low risk women? *Ultrasound Obstet Gynecol 15: 451-455.*

- **Benacerraf BR, Shipp TD & Bromley B (2006):** Three-dimensional US of the fetus: volume imaging. *Radiology 2006; 238(3):988-996.*

- **Benn A, Ying J, Beazoglou T & Egan JF (2001):** Estimates for the sensitivity and false-positive rates for second trimester serum screening for Down syndrome and trisomy 18 with adjustment for cross-identification and double positive results. *Prenat. Diagn. 21(1) 46.*

- **Benn A (2002):** Advances in prenatal screening for Down syndrome: I. General principles and second trimester testing. *Clinica Chimica Acta. 323: 1-16.*

162

- **Benn A (2002):** Advances in prenatal screening for Down syndrome: II first trimester testing, integrated testing, and future directions. *Clinica Chimica Acta. 324: 1-11.*

- **Benn PA, Fang M, Egan JFX, Horne D & Collins R (2003):** Incorporation of inhibin-A in second-trimester screeni for Down syndrome. *Obstet Gynecol 2003; 101:451-4.*

- **Benn P, Egan J, Fang M & Bindman R (2004):** Change in utilization of prenatal diagnosis. *The American College of Oobstetrician &Gynecologists.Obstetrics & Gynecology 2004; 103: 1255-1260.*

- **Bennett RL, Hart KA, O'Rourke E et al., (2002):** Fabry disease in genetic counseling practice: Recommendations of the National Society of Genetic Counselors. *J Genet Counsel. 2002; 11(2):121-146.*

- **Bennett RL, Motulsky AG, Bittles A et al., (2002):** Genetic counseling and screening of consanguineous couples and their offspring: Recommendations of the National Society of Genetic Counselors. *J Genet Counsel. 2002; 11(2):97-119.*

- **Bindra R, Heath V, Liao A, Spencer K & Nicolaides K (2002):** One- stop clinic for assessment of risk for trisomy 21 at 11-14 weeks: a prospective study of 15 030 pregnancies. *Ultrasound Obstet Gynecol 2002; 20: 219- 15.*

- **Bittles AH (2002):** Endogamy, consanguinity and community genetics. *J Genet 2002; 81:91-8.*

- **Bland JM & Altman DG (1986):** Statistical methouds for assessing agreement between two methouds of clinical measurement. *Lancet 1986; 1: 307-310.*

- **Bogart MH, Pandian MR & Jones OW (1987):** Abnormal maternal serum chorionic gonadotrophin levels in pregnancies with fetal chromosome abnormalities. *Prenat Diagn 1987; 7:623-30.*

- **Borrell A, Casals E, Fortuny A, Farre MT, Gonce A, Sanchez A et al., (2004):** First- trimester screening for trisomy 21 combining biochemistry and ultrasound at individually optimal gestational ages. An interventional study. *Prenat Diagn 2004; 24: 451- 5.*

- **Bower C, Ryan A & Rudy E (2001):** Ascertainment of pregnancies terminated because of birth defects: *effect on completeness of adding a new source of data. Teratology 2001; 63:23-25.*

- **Braithwaite D, Emery J, Walter F et al., (2006):** Psychological impact of genetic counseling for familial cancer: A systematic review and meta-analysis. *Fam Cancer. 2006; 5(1):61-75.*

163

- **Brambati B, Macintosh MC, Teisner B et al.**, **(1993):** Low maternal serum serum levels of pregnancy associated plasma protein A (PAPP-A) in the first trimester in association with abnormal fetal karyotype. *Br J Obstet Gynacol 100: 324.*

- **Braunstein GD, Rasor J, Danzer H et al.**, **(1976):** Serum human chorionic gonadotrophin levels throughout normal pregnancy. *Am. J. Obstet. Gynacol. 126: 678-681.*

- **Bromley B, Doubilet P, Frigoletto FD Jr, krauss C, Estroff JA & Benacerraf BR (1994):** Is fetal hyperechoic bowel on second trimester sonogram an indication for amniocentesis? *Obstet Gynecol 83: 647-51.*

- **Bromley B, Lieberman E, Laboda LA & Benacerraf BR (1995):** Echogenic intracardiac focus, a sonographic sign for Down syndrome? *Obstet Gynecol 86: 998-1001.*

- **Brown DL, Roberts DJ & Miller WA (1994):** Left ventricular echogenic focus in the fetal heart: pathologic correlation. *J Ulterasound Med 13: 613-6.*

- **Buckley S (2000):** Living with Down syndrome. Portsmouth, UK: The Down syndrome Educational Trust.

- **Burke C, Caulle A, Cinnsz S, Moss J, Pujol I, Scott I, Stallings J & Tomasin M (2006):** Wikipedia information about Down syndrome. This article is licensed under the GNU Free Documentation License. It uses material from the Wikipedia article "Down syndrome". *(Last updated: 2006 / last visit: December 4, 2006).*

- **Canick JA, Knight GJ, Palomaki GE et al.**, **(1988):** Second trimester maternal serum unconjugated oestriol in pregnancies with Down syndrome. *Br J Obstet Gynaecol 1988; 95:330-3.*

- **Canick JA & Saller DN (1993):** Maternal serum screening for aneuploidy and open fetal defects. *Obstetrics and Gynecology Clinics of Noth Americo 20: 443-454.*

- **Canick J, Lambert- Messerlian G, Palomaki G, Neveux L, Malone F, Ball R, Nuberg D, Comstock C, Bukowski R, Saade G & Berkowitz ZR (2008):**Comparison of serum markers in first- trimester Down Syndrome screening.*Obstet Gynecol 2008: 1192- 9.*

- **Chard T (1991):** Biochemistery and endocrinology of the Down syndrome pregnancy. *Ann. N. Y. Acad Sci. 626580-626596.*

- **Cicero S, Curcio P, Papagerorghiou A, Sonek J & Nicolaides K (2001):** Absence of the nasal bone in fetuses with trisomy 21 at 11-14 weeks of gestation: an observational study. *Lancent 2001; 358: 1665-7.*

- **Cicero S, Longo D, Rembouskos G, Sacchini C & Nicolaides KH (2003):** Absent nasal bone at 11-14 weeks of gestation and chromosomal defects. *Ultrasound Obstet Gynecol 2003; 22: 31-5.*

- **Cicero S, Sonek JD & Mckenna DS (2003):** nasal bone hypoplasia in trisomy 21 at 15-22 weeks gestation *Ultrasound Obstet. Gynecol 2003; 21: 15-8.*

- **Cicero S, Avgidou K, Rembouskos G, Kagan KO & Nicolaides KH (2006):** Nasal bone in first-trimester screening for trisomy 21.*Am J Obstet Gynecol 2006; 195: 109-14.*

- **Clericuzio (2001):** Prenatal dignosis/ screening procedures Vol 19; 2001.*Department of Pediatrics, the University of New Mexico, Albuquerque, NM, 87131. The Genetic Drift Newsletter is not copyrighted*

- **Cole LA, Rinne KM, Mahajan SM et al., (1999):** Urinary screening tests for fetal Down syndrome: I Fresh β-core fragment. *Prenat Diagn 19: 340-350.*

- **Cuckle HS & Wald NJ (1984):** Principles of screening. In: Wald NJ, editor. Antenatal and neonatal screening. Oxford: *Oxford University Press.*

- **Cuckle H, Densem J & Wald NJ (1994):** Repeat maternal serum testing in multiple markers Down syndrome screening programes. *Prenat Diagn 1994; 14:603– 607.* Prenatal screening for Down syndrome *May/June 2005 _ Vol. 7 _ No. 5 353*

- **Cuckle HS (2000):** Biochemical screening for Down syndrome. *European Journal of Obstetrics & Gynecology and Reproductive Biology 92: 97-101.*

- **Cuckle H (2001):** Integrating antenatal Down syndrome screening: *Curr Opin Obstet Gynecol. 13: 175-181.*

- **Cuckle H & Arbuzova S (2005):** Epidemiology of aneuploidy. In: Evans MI., editor. Prenatal diagnosis: genetics, reproductive risks, testing and management. *York, PA, USA: Techbooks; 2005.*

- **Cuckle H (2005):** Primary prevention of Down syndrome. *Int J Med Sci.july 1, 2005; 2(3): 93-99)(last visit: January 7, 2007).*

- **Cunniff C (2004):** Prenatal Screening and Diagnosis for Pediatricians. American Academy of Pediatrics. *Pediatrics vol.114 no. 3 September 2004, pp. 889-894.*

- **Cunningham FG, MacDonald PC, Gant NF, Leveno KJ, Gilstrap LC III, Hankins GDV et al., (1997):** Williams's obstetrics. 20th ed. Stamford, Connecticut: *Appleton & Lange, 1997.*

165

- **David T, Robert G, Diana W, Tracy B & John B (2000):** Six years Survey of screening for Down syndrome by maternal age and midtrimester ultrasound scan. *BMJ. 320: 606-10.*

- **Dourmishev A & Janniger (2003):** Down syndrome .e medicine 2003. *(Last updated: June 22, 2006 / last visit: January 7, 2007).*

- **Drugan A, Johnson MP & Evans MI (2000):** Ultrasound screening for fetal chromosome anomalies. *Am J Med Genet. 90: 98-107.*

- **Eddleman K, Berkowitz R, Kharbutli Y, Malone F, Viddaver J & Flint Porter T (2003):** Pregnancy loss rates after mid trimester amniocentesis: the FASTER trial. *Am J Obstet Gynecol 2003; 189(6):S111.*

- **Egan JF, Benn P, Borgida AF, Rodis JF, Campbell WA & Vintzlloes A (2000):** Efficacy of Screening for Fetal Down Syndrome in the United States From 1974 to 1997. The American College of Obstetricians and Gynecologists. *Obstet Gynecol 2000; 96(6): 979-85.*

- **Egan JFX, Malakh L, Turner G, Markenson G, Wax J, Benn PA (2001):** Role on ultrasound for Down syndrome screening of the advanced maternal age population. *Am J Obstet Gynecol. 185: 1028-31.*

- **Egan JF, Kaminsky LM, DeRoche ME, Barsoom MJ, Borgida AF & Benn PA (2002):** Antenatal Down syndrome screening in the united states in 2001: a survey of maternal- fetal medicine specialists. *Am J Obstet Gynecol 187, 1230- 1234.*

- **Eiben B, Bartels I, Bahr-Porsch S et al., (1990):** Cytogenetic analysis of 750 spontaneous abortions with the direct preparation method of chorionic villi and its implications for studying genetic causes of pregnancy wastage. *American Journal of Human Genetics 47: 656-663.*

- **Eiben B, Bartels I, Bahr-Porsch S et al., (1996):** Cytogenetic analysis of 750 spontaneous abortions with the direct preparation method of chorionic villi and its implications for studying genetic causes of pregnancy wastage. *American Journal of Human Genetics 47: 656-663.*

- **Faro C, Benoit B, Wegrzyn P, Chaoui R & Nicolaides KH (2005):** Three- dimensional sonographic description of the fetal frontal bones and metopic suture. *Ultrasound Obstet Gynecol 2005; 26: 618-621.*

- **Fenech M, Aitken C & Folate R (1998):** vitamin B12, homocysteine status and DNA damage in young Australian adults. *Carcinogenesis 1998; 19:1163-1171.*

- **Filly RA (2000):** Obstetrical sonography: the best way to terrify a pregnant woman. *J Ultrasound Med 19: 1-5.*

- **Freeman SB, Yang Q, Allran K et al., (2000):** Women with a reduced ovarian complement may have an increased risk for a child with Down syndrome. *Am. J. Hum. Genet, 66, 1680–1683.*

- **Fung Kee Fung K, Eason E, Crane J, Armson A, De La Ronde S & Farine D (2003):** SOCG Clinical Practic Guidelines. Prevention of RH Alloimmunization. *J Obstet Gynaecol Can 2003; 25(9):765-73.*

- **Gale T (2006):** Prenatal diagnosis techniques.*Thomson Gale, a part of the Thomson Corporation. Copyright 2006.*

- **Geipel A, Berg C, Katalinic A, Ludwig M, Germer U, Diedrich K & Gembruch U (2004):** *different Preferences for Prenatal diagnosis in pregnancies following assisted reproduction versus spontaneous conception. **Reprod Biomed Online 8, 119 – 124.***

- **Genetic & public policy center (2007):** prenatal diagnosis.

- **George T & Capone M (2001):** Down syndrome: Advances in Molecular Biology and the Neurosciences. *Developmental and Behavioral Pediatrics 22:40-59.*

- **Giacherio D (2002):** Prenatal screening for Down syndrome. *M labs spectrum department of pathology, vol 16, no. 3, July 2002.*

- **Gissler M, Klemetti R, Sevon T & Hemminki E (2004):** Monitoring of IVF birth outcomes in Finland: a data quality study. *BMC Med Inform Decis Mak 4, 3.*

- **Graves C, Miller K & Sellers A (2002):** Maternal Serum Triple Analyte Screening in Pregnancy University of Tennessee College of Medicine. *The American Academy of Family Physicians.*

- **Green JM (1994):** Women's experiences of prenatal screening and diagnosis. In: Abramsky L, Chapple J, eds. prenatal diagnosis: the human side. *New York: Chapman & Hall, 1994:37-53.*

- **Hackshaw AK, Kennard A & Wald NJ (1995):** Detection of pregnancies with trisomy 18 in screening programmes for Down syndrome. *Journal of Medical Screening 2: 228-229.*

- **Hackshaw AK & Wald NJ (2001):** Repeat testing in antenatal screening for Down syndrome using dimeric inhibin-A in combination with other maternal serum markers. *Prenat Diagn 2001; 21:58-61.*

167

- **Haddow JE, Knight GJ, Kloza EM & Palomaki GE (1986):** Alpfa-fetoprotein, vaginal bleeding and pregnancy risk. *Br J Obstet Gynaecol. 93: 589-93.*

- **Haddow JE, Palomaki GE, Knight GJ et al., (1992):** Prenatal screening for Down syndrome with use of maternal serum markers. *N. Engl. J. Med. 327: 588-593.*

- **Haddow JE, Palomaki GE, Knight GJ, Cunningham GC, Lustig LS & Boyd PA (1994):** Reducing the need for amniocentesis in women 35 years of age or older with serum markers for screening. *N Engl J Med 1994; 330:1114-8.*

- **Haddow JE, Palomaki GE, Knight GJ, Foster DL & Neveux LM (1998):** Second trimester screening for Down syndrome using maternal serum dimeric inhibin. *A J Med Screen 1998; 5:115–119.*

- **Haddow JE, Palomaki GE, Knight GJ & Canick JA (2004):** Prenatal Screening for Major Fetal Disorders: *The Foundation for Blood Research Handbook, Volume II: Screening for Down syndrome. 1998. Accessed October 26, 2004.*

- **Hallahan T, Krantz D, Orlandi F et al., (2000):** First trimester biochemical screening for Down syndrome: free beta hCG versus intact hCG. *Prenat Diagn 20: 785-9.*

- **Hampel H, Sweet K, Westman JA et al., (2004):** Referral for cancer genetics consultation: A review and compilation of risk assessment criteria. *J Med Genet. 2004; 41(2):81-91.*

- **Hassold T & Sherman S (2000):** Down syndrome: genetic recombination and the origin of the extra chromosome 21. *Clin. Gent. 57. 95-100.*

- **Hassold T & Hunt (2001):** The genesis of human aneuploidy. *Nat Rev Genet 2001; 2:280-291.*

- **Hattori M, Fujiyama A & Taylor T (2000):** The DNA sequence of human chromosome 21: *Nature 405: 311-319.*

- **Hecht CA & Hook EB (1996):** Rates of Down syndrome at live birth by one year maternal age intervals in studies with apparent close to complete ascertainment in populations of European origin: A proposed revised rate schedule for use in genetic and prenatal screening. *Am. J. of Med. Genet. 62: 376-385.*

- **Hobbs CA, Sherman SL, Yi P, Hopkins SE, Torfs CP, Hine RJ, Pogribna M, Rozen R & James SJ (2000):** Polymorphisms in genes involved in folate metabolism as maternal risk factors for Down syndrome. *Am J Hum Genet 2000; 67:623-630.*

- **Holding S (1997):** Biochemical screening for Down syndrome in the second trimester of pregnancy. *PhD thesis, University of Hull, UK.*

- **Holding S (2002):** Current state of screening for Down syndrome. *Ann Clin Biochom 39:1-11.*

- **Hook EM (1981):** Rates of chromosome abnormalities at different maternal ages. *Obstet. Gynecol., 58:282*

- **Huang T, Watt HC & Wald NJ (1997):** The effect of differences in the distribution of maternal age on England and Wales on the performance of prenatal screening for Down syndrome. *Prenat Diagn 97; 17: 615- 21.*

- **Hyett J, Moscoso G & Nicolaides K (1997):** Abnormalities of the heart and great arteries in first trimester chromosomally abnormal fetuses. *Am J Med Genet. 69: 207-16.*

- **Jain VK, Nalini P, Chandra R & Srinivasan S (1993):** Congenital malformations, reproductive wastage and consanguineous mating. *Aust NZ J Obstet Gynaecol 1993; 33:33-6.*

- **Jaques AM, Collins VR, Haynes K, Sheffield LJ, Francis I, Forbes R & Halliday JL (2006):** Using record linkage and manual follow-up to evaluate the Victorian maternal serum screening quadruple test for Down syndrome, trisomy 18 and neural tube defects. *J Med Screen. 2006; 13 (1): 8 -13.*

- **Jaques AM, Halliday JL, Francis I, Bonacquisto L, Forbes R, Cronin A & Sheffield LJ (2007):** Follow up and evaluation of the Victorian first- trimester combined screening program for Down syndrome and trisomy 18. *BJOG 2007; 114: 812- 818.*

- **Jauniaux E & Burton GJ (1992):** The effect of smoking in pregnancy on early placental morphology. *Obstet Gynecol. 79:645-648.*

- **Jill Mauldin (2000):** Prenatal Diagnosis and fetal therapy- What lies in future? *Indian J Pediatr. 67: (12): 899-905.*

- **Kaminsky L, Egan J, Ying J, Bgorgida A, DeRoche M & Benn P (2001):** Combined second trimester biochemical and ultrasound screening for Down syndrome is highly effective. *Am J Obstet Gynecol. 185: S78.*

- **Kandinov L (2005):** Periconceptional exposure to oral contraceptive pills and risk for Down syndrome. *Medscape Ob/Gyn & women's health. 2005; 10, 1.*

- **Knight PG, Muttukrishna S & Groome NP (1996):** Development and application of a two-site enzyme immunoassay for the determination of "total" activin-A concentrations in serum and follicular fluid. *J Endocrinol 148: 267-279.*

- **Knight GJ & Palomaki GE (2003):** Epidemiologic monitoring of prenatal screening for neural tube defects and Down syndrome. *Clin Lab Med 2003; 22:531–551.*

- **Kumar S & O'Brien A (2004):** Recent developments in fetal medicine. *BMJ 2004; 328: 1002-1006 (24 April), doi: 10, 1136/ bmj. 328, 7446.1002* center for fetal care, queen charlotte's and Chelsea hospital, imperial collage landon.

- **Lapunzina P, Camelo L, Rittler M & Castilla E (2002):** Risks of congenital anomalies in large for gestational age infants. *J Pediatric 2002; 140: 200-204.*

- **Lejeune J (2006):** *(Retrieved on 2006-06-02).*

- **Leshin L (2007):** Prenatal diagnosis for Down syndrome. ACOG practice Bulletin. Screening for fetal chromosomal abnormalities. *Obstet Gynacol. 109(1), Jan 2007.*

- **Lilford RJ (1997):** Commentary: Down syndrome and parity. *BMJ 1997; 314:721.*

- **Macri JN, Kasturi RV, Krantz DA, Cook EJ, Sunderji SG & Larsen JW (1990):** Maternal serum Down syndrome screening: unconjugated oestriol is not useful. *Am J Obstet Gynacol. 162:672-3.*

- **Malone FD & D'Alton ME (2003):** First-trimester sonographic screening for Down syndrome. *Obstet Gynecol 2003; 102:1066-79.*

- **Malone FD, Wald NJ, Canick JA, Ball RH, Nyberg DA, Comstock CH et al., (2003):** First and second- trimester evaluation of risk (FASTER) trial: Principle results of the NICHID multicenter Down syndrome screening study. *Am J Obstet Gynecol 2003; 189: s 56.*

- **Malone FD, Canick JA, Ball RH, Nyberg DA, Comstock CH, Bukowski R et al., (2005):** First or second- trimester screening, or both, for Down syndrome. *N Engl J Med 2005; 353: 2001- 11.*

- **Malone FD, Cuckle H, Ball RH, Nyberg DA, Comstock CH, Saade G, Berkowitz RL, Gross SJ, Dugoff L & Craigo SD (2005b):** Contigent screening for tisomy 21-results from a general population screening trial. *Am J Obstet Gynecol 193, S 29.*

- **Maymon R, Jauniaux E, Holmes A, Wiener YM, Dreazen E & Herman A (2001):** Nuchal translucency measurement and pregnancy outcome after assisted conception versus spontaneously conceived twins. *Hum Reprod 16, 1999-2004.*

170

- **Maymon R & Shulman A (2004):** Integrated first- and second trimester Down syndrome screening test among unaffected IVF pregnancies. *Prenat Diagn 24, 125- 129.*

- **Maymon R, Neeman O, Shulman A, Rosen H & Herman A (2005):** Current concepts of Down syndrome screening tests in assisted reproduction twin pregnancies: another double trouble. *Prenat Diag 25, 746-50.*

- **McKusick V (1999):** Online Mendelian Inheritance in Man (OMIM). *Baltimore, MD, Center for Medical Genetics, Johns Hopkins University and Bethesda, MD, National Center for Biotechnology Information, National Library of Medicine.*

- **Meier C, Huang T, Wyatt PR & Summers AM (2002):** Accuracy of expected risk of Down syndrome using the second-trimester triple test. *Clin Chem 2002; 48:653-655.*

- **Merkatz IK, Nitowsky HM, Macri JN et al., (1984):** An association between low maternal serum alpha-fetoprotein and fetal chromosome abnormalities. *Am J Obstet Gynecol 1984; 148:886-94.*

- **Meyers C, Adam R, Dungan J & Prenger V (1997):** Aneuploidy in twin gestation: When is maternal age advanced? *Obstet Gynecol 89, 248-251.*

- **MFMER (2006):** Down syndrome: Screening and diagnosis. Mayo foundation for medical education research.

- **MFMER (2007):** Down syndrome. Mayo foundation for medical education and research. *(Last updated :2007 /last visit: January 11, 2007).*

- **Montfrans JM, Dorland M & Oosterhuis GJ et al., (1999):** Increased concentrations of follicle-stimulating hormone in mothers of children with Down syndrome. *Lancet, 353, 1853–1854.* New Guidelines Recommend Universal Prenatal Screening for Down Syndrome CME/CE

- **Montfrans, Lambalk, Von Holf & Van Vugt (2001):** Are elevated FSH concentrations in the preconceptional period a risk factor for Down syndrome pregnancies. *Human Reproducton, vol. 16, no. 6, 1276-1273, June 2001.*

- **Morris JK, Mutton DE, Alberman E et al. (2002):** Revised estimates of maternal age specific live birth prevalence of Down syndrome in the absence of antenatal screening and selective termination. *J Med Screen 2002; 9:2-6.*

- **Mueller RF & Young ID (2001):** Elements of Medical Genetics. *11th Edn. Edinburgh: Churchill Livingstone; 2001. p. 100/245.*

- **Muller F, Dreux S, Lemeur a, Sault C, Desgres J, Bernard MA, Giorgetti C, Lemay C, Mirallie S & Beauchet A (2003):** Medically assisted reproduction and second-trimester maternal marker screening for Down syndrome. *Prenat Diagn 23, 1073-1076.*

- **Nasseri A, Mukherjee T, Grifo J.A et al., (1999):** Elevated day 3 serum follicle stimulating hormone and/or estradiol may predict fetal aneuploidy. *Fertil. Steril; 71, 715–718.*

- **Nazario B (2003):** Dad's age raises Down syndrome risk too. *Web MD Medical News.*

- **Newberger D (2000):** Down syndrome: Prenatal Risk Assessment and Diagnosis. *Am Fam Physician 2000; 62:825-32,837-8.).*State University of New York at Buffalo, Buffalo, New York *(last visit: december 4, 2006).*

- **Newby D, Aitken DA, Crossky JA, Howatson AG, Macri JN & Connor JM (1997):** Biochemical markers of trisomy 21 and the pathophysiology of Down syndrome pregnancies. *Prenat Diagn 17: 941-951.*

- **Newby D, Aitken DA, Howatson AG & Connor JM (2000):** Placental synthesis of oestriol in Down syndrome pregnancies. *Placenta. 21:263-7.*

- **Nicolaides KH, Azar G, Byrene D, Mansur C & Marks k (1992):** Fetal nuchal translucency: ultrasound screening for chromosomal defects in first trimester of pregnancy. *Bmj 1992; 302: 867-89.*

- **Nicolaides KH (2003):** Screening for chromosomal defects ultrasound. *Obstet & Gynecol 2003; 21: 313-21.*

- **Nicolaides KH (2004):** Nuchal translucency and other first- trimester sonographic markers of chromosomal abnormalities. *Am J Obstet Gynecol 2004; 191: 45- 67.*

- **Nicolaides K, Spencer K, Avgidou K, Faiola S & Falcon O (2005):** Multicenter study of first trimester screening for trisomy 21 in 75 821 pregnancies: results and estimation of the potential impact of individual risk- orientated two- stage first- trimester screening. *Ultrasound Obestet Gynecol 2005; 25: 211- 6.*

- **Nicolaides k (2006):** Patient information- first trimester screening for Down syndrome. Fetal medicine center. *(Retrieved on: 2006/ last modified: 2008 Jan., wikipedia).*

- **Niemimaa M, Heinoen S, Seppala M, Hippelainen M, Martikmainen H & Rynanen M (2001):** First trimester screening for Down syndrome in vitro fertilization pregnancies. *Fertil Steril 76, 1282- 1283.*

- **NSC (2001):** National screening committee. Antenatal Screening service for Down syndrome in England (2001). A report to UK. Augest 2002. **UK National screening committee programer directorate2002.**

- **Nyberg DA, Resta RC, Mahony BS, Dubinsky T, Luthy DA, Hickok DE & Luthardt FW (1993):** Fetal hyperechogenic bowl and Down syndrome. *Ultrasound Obstet Gynecol 3: 330-3.*

- **Nyberg DA, Luthy DA, Resta RG, Nyberg BC & Williams MA (1998):** Age-adjusted ultrasound risk assessment for fetal Down syndrome during the second trimester: description of the method and analysis of 142 cases. *Ultrasound Obstet Gynecol 12: 8-14.*

- **Nyberg DA, Souter VL, El-Bastawissi A, Young S, Luthardt F & Luthy DA (2001):** Isolated sonographic markers for detection of Down syndrome in the second trimester of pregnancy. *J Ultrasound Med. 20: 1053-63.*

- **Oddens BJ, Tonkelaar I & Nieuwenhuyse H (1999):** Psychological experiences in women facing fertility problems- a comparative survey. *Hum Reprod 14, 255-261.*

- **O'leary P, Breheny N, Dickinson J, Bower C, Goldblatt J, Hewitt B, Murch A & Stock R (2006):** First -trimester combined screening for Down syndrome and other fetal anomalies. *Obstet Gynecol 2006; vol.107: 869 – 876.*

- **Orlandi F, Rossi C, Orlandi E, Jakil MC, Hallahan TW, Macri VJ & Krantz DA (2005):** first-trimester screening for trisomy 21 using a simplified method to assess the presence or absence of the fetal nasal bone. *Am J Obstet Gynecol 2005; 192: 1107-11.*

- **Ormond KE, Pergament E & Fine BA (1996):** Pre-screening education in multiple marker screening programs: the effect on patient anxiety and knowledge. *J Genetic Counseling 5: 69-80.*

- **Otano L, Aiello H, Igarzabal L, Matayoshi T & Gadow EC (2002):** Association between first trimester absence of fetal nasal bone on ultrasound and Down syndrome. *Prenat Diagn 2002; 22: 930-2.*

- **Ozturk M, Bellet D, Manil L, Hennen G, Frydman R & Wands J (1987):** Physiological studies on human chorionic gonadotrophin (hCG), α-hCG and β-hCG as measured by specific monoclonal immunoradiometric assays. *Endocrinol 120:549-58.*

- **Palomaki CE, Knight GJ, McCarthy JE, Haddow JE & Donhowe JM (1995):** Maternal serum screening for Down syndrome in the United States: a survey. *Am J Obstet Gynecol 1997; 176: 1046-51.*

- **Palomaki GE, Neveux LM & Haddow JE (1995):** Are DADs (discriminant aneuploidy detection) as good as MoMs (multiples of the median)? *Am J Obstet Gynecol 1995; 173:1895–6.*

- **Palomaki G, Bradley L & McDowell G (2005):** Technical standards and guidelines: Prenatal screening for Down syndrome. *ACMG Laboratory Quality Assurance Committee. May/June 2005 _ Vol. 7 _ No. 5.*

- **Palomaki G, Bradley L & McDowell G (2006):** Technical Standards and Guidelines: Prenatal Screening for Down syndrome. *AMERICAN COLLEGE OF MEDICAL GENETICS Standards and Guidelines for Clinical Genetics Laboratories 2006 Edition.*

- **Pandya A (2006):** Screening for Down syndrome. *J Obstet Gynecol India vol. 56, no. 3: May/June 2006 pg 205-211.* University college Landon hospitals, London, England (UK).

- **Papp C, Beke A, Mezei G, Toth-Pal E & Papp Z (2002):** Chorionic Villus sampling: a15 year experience. *Fetal Diagn Ther 2002; 17:218-27.*

- **Patterson D (1995):** The integrated map of human chromosome 21. In etiology and pathogenesis of Down syndrome. *Wiley-Liss. P 43-55.*

- **Penrose LS (1961):** Mongolism. *Br Med Bull 1961; 17: 184-9.*

- **Plasencia W, Dagklis T, Sotiriadis A, Borenstein M & Nicoladies KH (2007):** Frontomaxillary facial angle at 11+ 0 to 13+ 6 weeks gestation- reproducibility of measurements. *Ultrasound Obstet Gynecol 2007; 29: 18- 21.*

- **Qu J & Thomas K (1995):** Inhibin and activin production in human placenta. *Endocr Rev 16: 485-507.*

- **Raty R, Anttila L, Virtanen A, Koskinen P, Laitinen P, Morsky P, Tiitinen A, Martikainen H & Ekblad U (2003):** Maternal midtrimester free beta- HCG and AFP serum levels in spontaneous singleton pregnancies complicated by gestational diabetes mellitus, pregnancy- induced hypertension or obstetric cholestasis. *Prenat Diagn 23, 1045-1048.*

- **Ray J, Meier C, Vermeulen MJ, Boss S, Wyatt PR & Cole DEC (2002):** Association of neural tube defects and folic acid food fortification. *Lancet 2002; 360:2047–2048.*

- **Ray J, Meier C, Vermeulen M, Cole D & Wyatt P (2003):** Unchanged Prevalence of Trisomy 21 With Folic Acid Food Fortification in Canada.

- **Reynolds TM, Nix AB, Dunstan FD & Dawson AJ (1993):** Age-specific detection and false-positive rates: an aid to counseling in Down syndrome risk screening. *Obstet Gynecol 1993; 81:447-50.*

- **Rice JD, Mcintosh SF & Halstead AC (2005):** Second- trimester maternal serum screening for Down syndrome in vitro fertilization pregnancies. *Prenat Diagn 25, 234-238.*

- **Rose P, Kim H, Augustine E & Edwards K (2003):** Parity and the Risk of Down syndrome. *Am J Epidemiol 2003; 158:503-508.*

- **Saenz RB (1999):** Primary care of infants and young children with Down syndrome. *Am Fam Physician 1999; 59:381-90,392,395-6.*

- **Saller DN & Canick JA (1996):** Maternal serum screening for fetal Down syndrome: clinical aspects. *Clin. Obstet. Gynecol. 39(4): 783-792.*

- **Saltvedt S, Almstrom H, Kublickas M, Valentin L & Grunewald C (2006):** Detection of malformations in chromosomally normal fetuses by routine ultrasound at 12 to 18 weeks of gestation – a randomised controlled trial in 39572 pregnancies. *BJOG 2006; 113: 664 - 674.*

- **Sancken U & Bartels I (2001):** Biochemical screening for chromosomal disorders and neural tube defects (NTD): is adjustment of maternal alpha-fetoprotein (AFP) still appropriate in insulin-dependent diabetes (IDDM). *Prenat Diagn, 2001; 21:383-386.*

- **Sara Cate (1999):** Multiple markers screening for Down syndrome- Whom should we screen? *J Am Board FAM Pract. 12: 367-374*

- **Scheffer GJ, Broekmans FJ, Dorland M et al., (1999):** Antral follicle counts by transvaginal ultrasonography are related to age in women with proven natural fertility. *Fertil. Steril; 72, 845–851.*

- **Schon EA, Kim S, Ferreira J C, Magalhaes P, Grace M, Warburton D & Gross S (2000):** Chromosomal non-disjunction in human oocytes: Is there a mitochondrial connection? *Human Reproduction 15 (2) 160-172.*

- **Sebire NJ, Snijders RJ, Hughes K, Sepulveda W & Nicolaides KH (1996):** Screening for trisomy 21 in twin pregnancies by maternal age and fetal nuchal translucency thickness at 10- 14 weeks of gestation. *Br J Obstet Gynecol 191, 999-1003.*

- **Sepulveda W, Wong A & Dezerega V (2007):** First- Trimester Ultrasonographic screening for Trisomy 21 Using Fetal Nuchal Translucency and Nasal Bone. *Obstetrics & Gynecology vol. 109, no.5, May 2007.*

- **Shafi B, Kaleem M, Hafi S, Sistrom C, Coombs B, Reuter k, Krasny R & Lin E (2007):** Down syndrome, prenatal finidings. *Department of Radiology, Royal Liverpool Children's NHS Trust HospitalOrthopedic Center,UK.*

- **Sherod C, Sebire NJ, Soares W et al., (1997):** Prenatal diagnosis of trisomy 18 at 10-14 week ultrasound scans. *Ultrasound Obstet Gynacol 10: 387-390.*

- **Shire B (2005):** Bright Beginnings: A Guide for New Parents. Down syndrome Research Foundation UK.

- **Simpson JL (2005):** Choosing the best prenatal screening protocol. *N Engi J Med 353, 2068-2070.*

- **Singh D, Sing J, Cibis G, Talavera F, James J, Brown L & Roy H (2005):** Prenatal Diagnosis for Congenital Malformations and Genetic Disorders. *e medicine, (Last Updated: january 23, 2006 / last visit: november 18, 2006).*

- **Smith-Bindman R, Hosmer W, Feldstein VA, Deeks J & Goldberg JD (2001):** Second trimester ultrasound to detect fetuses with Down syndrome: a meta-analysis. *JAMA. 285: 1044-55.*

- **Smith-Bindman R, Chu P, Bacchetti P, Waters JJ, Mutton D & Alberman E (2003):** Prenatal screening for Down syndrome in England and Wales and population-based birth outcomes. *Am J Obstet Gynecol 2003; 189:980-5.*

- **Snoek J, Borenstein M, Dagklis T, Persico N & Nicolaides KH (2006):** Fronto maxillary facial angle in fetuses with trisomy 21 at 11-13+6 weeks. *Am J Obstet Gynecol 2006.*

- **Snoek J, Borenstein M, Dagklis T, Persico N & Nicoladies KH (2007):** Frontomaxillary facial angle in fetuses with trisomy 21 at 11- 13th weeks. *American Journal of Obstetrics & Gynecology 2007; 196: 271.e 1- 271. e4.*

- **Souka AP, Von Kssenberg CS, Hyett JA, Snoek JD & Nicolaides KH (2005):** Increased nuchal translucency with normal karyotype. *Am J Obstet Gynecol 2005; 192: 1005; 21.*

- **Souter VL, Nyberg DA, El-Bastawissi A, Zebelman A, Luthhardt F & Luthy DA (2002):** Correlation of ultrasound findings and biochemical markers in the second trimester of pregnancy in fetuses with trisomy 21. *Prenat Diagn. 22: 175-82.*

176

- **Spencer K (1998):** The influence of smoking on maternal serum AFP and free beta hCG levels and the impact on screening for Down syndrome. *Prenat Diagn 1998; 18:225.*

- **Spencer K, Berry E, Crossley JA, Aitken DA & Nicolaides KH (2000):** Is maternal serum total hCG a marker of trisomy 21 in the first trimester of pregnancy? *Prenat Diagn 20: 311-7.*

- **Spencer K & Nicolaides KH (2003):** Screening for trisomy 21 in twins using first trimester ultra sound and maternal serum biochemistry in a one- stop clinic: a review of three years experience. *BJOG 110, 276-280.*

- **Stein MT, Scioscia A, Jones KL, Cohen WI, Glass CK & Glass RF (1997):** Responding to parental concerns after a prenatal diagnosis of trisomy 21. *J Dev Behav Pediatr 1997; 18:42-6.*

- **Tabor A, Philip J, Madsen M, Bang J, Obel EB & Pedersen N (1987):** Randomised controlled trial of genetic amniocentesis in 4606 low-risk women. *Lancet 1987; 1:1287–93.*

- **Taketa K (1995):** Oncofetal alterations of AFP sugar chains. *Jpn J Electrophoresis. 39: 133-6.*

- **Tietz NW (1999):** Maternal and fetal health assessment. In: *Textbook of Clinical Chemistry; 3rd ed., Greene MF, Fencl MD, and Tulchinsky D, Eds. Philadelphia, W.B. Saunders, p. 1742.*

- **Toth-Pal E, Papp C, Beke A, Ban Z & Papp Z (2004):** Genetic amniocentesis in multiple pregnancies. *Fetal Diagn Ther 2004; 19:138-44.*

- **Tul N, Spencer K, Noble P, Chan C & Nicolaides K (1999):** Screening for trisomy 18 by fetal nuchal translucency and maternal serum free beta- hCG and PAPP- A at 10-14 weeks of gestation. *Prenat Diagn 1999; 19: 1035- 42.*

- **Tunç M (2007):** Contemporary screening in pregnancy. *J Turkish – German Gynecol Assoc, vol.8 (3); 2007: 331-338.*

- **Verma IC, Prema A & Puri RK (1992):** Health Effects of Consanguinity in Pondicherry. *Indian J Ped 1992; 29:685- 92.*

- **Vintzileos AM & Egan JFX (1995):** Adjusting the risk for trisomy 21 on the basis of second-trimester ultrasonography. *Am J Obstet Gynecol 172: 837-44.*

- **Vintzileos AM, Campbell WA, Guzman ER et al., (1997):** Second-trimester ultrasound markers for detection of trisomy 21: which markers are best? *Obstet Gynecol 1997; 89: 941-4.*

177

- Wald N, Cuckle H, Densem J, Kennard A & Smith D (1992): Maternal serum screening for Down syndrome: The effect of routine ultrasound scans determination of gestational age and adjustement for maternal weight. *Br J Obstet Gynecol 1992; 99: 144-9.*

- Wald NJ & Kennard A (1992): Antenatal maternal serum screening for Down syndrome: results of a demonstration project. *BMJ 305: 391-394.*

- Wald NJ, Stone R, Cuckle HS et al., (1992): First trimester concentrations of PAPP-A and placental protein 14 in Down syndrome. *British Medical Journal 305: 28.*

- Wald NJ, Densen JW et al., (1994): Maternal serum free B-hCG in twin's pregnancies: implications for screening for Down syndrome. *Prenat Diagn 14:319-320.*

- Wald NJ, Kennard A & Hackshw AK (1995): First trimester serum screening for Down syndrome. *Prenat Diagn 15: 1227-40.*

- Wald NJ, Watt HC et al., (1996): Serum markers for Down syndrome in relation to number of previous births and maternal age. *Prenat Diagn 16: 699-703.*

- Wald NJ, Watt HC & George L (1996): Maternal serum inhibin A in pregnancies with insulin dependent diabetes mellitus: implication for screening fore Down syndrome. *Prenat Diagn 16: 923-6.*

- Wald NJ, Densem JW, George L, Muttukrishna S, Knight PG, Watt H et al., (1997): Inhibin- A in Down syndrome pregnancies: revised estimate of standard deviation. *Prenat Diagn 1997; 17:285–290.*

- Wald NJ. Kennard A, Hacskshaw AK & McGuire A (1997): A antenatal screening for Down syndrome. *Journal of Medical Screening 4:181-246.*

- Wald NJ, Huttly WJ & Hennessy CF (1999): Down syndrome screening in the UK in 1998. *lancet 354:1264.*

- Wald NJ, Watt HC & Hackshaw AK (1999): Integrated screening for Down syndrome on the basis of test performed during the first and second trimesters. *N. Engl. J. Med., 341, 461-467.*

- Wald NJ, White N, Morris JK, Huttly WJ & Canick JE (1999): Serum markers for Down syndrome in women who have had in vitro fertilization: implications for antenatal screening. *Br J Obstet Gynaecol 106, 1304-1306.*

- **Wald NJ, Hackshaw AH & Watt HC (2000):** Nuchal translucency and trisomy 18. *Prenatal Diagnosis 20: 353-357.*

- **Wald NJ, Hackshaw AK & George LM (2000):** Assay precision of serum alpha fetoprotein in antenatal screening for neural tube defects and Down syndrome. *J Med Screen 2000; 7:74 –77.*

- **Wald NJ & Hackshaw AK (2000):** Advances antenatal screening for Down syndrome. *Clin Obstet Gynecol 14; 4:563-580*

- **Wald NJ, Rish S & Hackshaw AK (2003):** Combining nuchal translucency and serum markers in prenatal screening for Down syndrome in twin pregnancies. *Prenat Diagn 23, 588- 592.*

- **Wald NJ, Rodeck C & Hackshaw AK et al., (2003):** SURUSS Research Group. First and second trimester antenatal screening for Down syndrome: the results of the Serum, Urine and Ultrasound Screening Study (SURUSS). *Health Technol Assess 2003; 7:1-77.*

- **Wald NJ, Rodeck C, Hackshaw AK & Rudnicka A (2004):** SURUSS in perspective. *BJOG 2004; 111: 521-531.*

- **Watt HC, Wald NJ & George L (1996):** Maternal serum inhibin-A levels in twin pregnancies: implications for screening for Down syndrome. *Prenat Diagn 1996; 16: 927–929.*

- **Weisz B & Rodeck C (2006):** An update on antenatal screening for Down syndrome and specific implications for assisted reproduction pregnancies. *Human Reproduction Update, vol. 12, no.5 pp.13-518.*

- **Weisz B, Pandya P, Chitty L, Jones P, Huttly W, Rodeck C et al., (2007):** Practical issues drawn from the implementation of the integrated test for Down syndrome screening into routine clinical practice. *BJOG 2007; 114: 493 – 497.*

- **Wellesley D, Boyle T, Barber J & Howe DT (2002):** Retrospective audit of different antenatal screening policies for Down syndrome in eight district general hospitals in one health region. *BMJ. 2002; 325(7354):15.*

- **Westergaad JG, Chemnitz J, Teisner B et al., (1983):** Pregnancy-associated plasma protein-A: A possible marker in the classification and prenatal diagnosis of Cornelia de Lange syndrome. *Prenat Diagn. 3: 225.*

- **Wilson R, Davies G, Gagnon A, Desiletes V, Reid G, Summer S, Wyatt P, Allen V & Langlois S (2005):** Amended Canadian guideline for prenatal diagnosis(2005) change to 2005-techniques for prenatal diagnosis. *J Obstet Gynaecol Can 2005; 27(11):1048-1054.*

- **Wojdemann KR, Larsen SO, Shalmi A, Sundberg K, Christiensen M & Tabor A (2001):** First trimester screening for Down syndrome and assisted reproduction: no basis for concern. *Prenat Diagn 21, 563- 565.*

- **Wojdemann K, Shalmi A, Christiansen M, Larsen S, Sundberg K, Brocks V et al., (2005):** Improved first- trimester Down syndrome screening performance by lowering the false positive rate: a prospective study of 9941 low- risk women. *Ultrasound Obstet Gynecol 2005; 25: 227- 33.*

- **Wood D (2006):** Down syndrome Laurance Frisch EBSCO. *BLUM patient and family learning center.*

- **Yamamoto R, Azuma M, Hoshi N, Kishida T, Satomura S & Fujimoto S (2001):** *Lens culinaris* agglutinin-reactive α-fetoprotein, an alternative variant to α-fetoprotein in prenatal screening for Down syndrome. *Human Reproduction, Vol. 16, No. 11, 2438-2444.*

- **Yaron Y & Mashiach R (2001):** Frist- trimester biochemical screening for Down syndrome. *Metabolic and Genetic Screening. 28: 2; 321-331.*

- **Zuckoff M (2002):** Choosing Naia a family's Journey. *New York: Beacan press.*

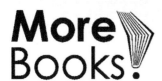
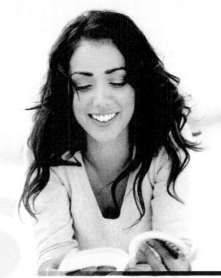